GENERAL ANAESTHESIA AND SEDATION IN DENTISTRY

A DENTAL PRACTITIONER HANDBOOK
SERIES EDITED BY DONALD D. DERRICK DDS LDS RCS

GENERAL ANAESTHESIA AND SEDATION IN DENTISTRY

C. M. HILL
BDS (Bris), FDS RCS(Ed)
*Lecturer in Oral Surgery,
Department of Dental Surgery,
School of Dentistry,
University of Leeds*

and

P. J. MORRIS
MB ChB, DObst, RCOG, FFARCS
*Lecturer in Anaesthesia,
Department of Anaesthesia,
University of Leeds*

WRIGHT·PSG
BRISTOL · LONDON · BOSTON
1983

© **John Wright & Sons Ltd**, 1983

All Rights Reserved. No part of this publication may be reproduced, stored in a retrieval system, or transmitted in any form or by any means, electronic, mechanical, photocopying, recording or otherwise, without the prior permission of the Copyright owner.

Published by
John Wright & Sons Ltd, 823–825 Bath Road, Bristol BS4 5NU, England
John Wright PSG Inc., 545 Great Road, Littleton, Massachusetts 01460, USA

British Library Cataloguing in Publication Data

Hill, C. M.
   General anaesthesia and sedation in dentistry.
   —(A Dental practitioner handbook; No. 32)
   1. Anaesthesia in dentistry
   I. Title   II. Morris, P. J.   III. Series
   617'.9676   RK510

ISBN 0 7236 0759 1

Library of Congress Catalog Card Number: 83-50556

Typeset and printed in Great Britain by
John Wright & Sons (Printing) Ltd at The Stonebridge Press, Bristol BS4 5NU

PREFACE

It has been our aim in writing this book to produce a concise and readable account of general anaesthesia and sedation as it relates to the practice of dentistry. Building on the basis of physiology and pharmacology acquired during the undergraduate course, we have provided a suitable summary of the scientific and practical aspects of dental anaesthesia. It is aimed primarily at the student, both in the clinic and in the final examination of the Bachelor of Dental Surgery, but it is also suitable for practitioners who may wish to refresh their knowledge and keep abreast of this expanding field.

The dangers of airway obstruction have been emphasized at the risk of repetition but it is our belief that this is the most serious complication of dental anaesthesia. Wherever possible we have attempted to build from the most basic level of knowledge, not to patronize but to ensure that the principles of treatment are understood at least as well as the practical details of such treatment.

The increased awareness of the general public and the changing nature of dental anaesthesia and sedation ensure that there is a wealth of material from which this book is drawn. There has been no attempt to produce a comprehensive treatise but we have included enough theoretical and practical instruction to give a basic, but thorough, understanding of this subject. A short bibliography is also included as an appendix for those who may wish to pursue their interest to a deeper level.

C. M. H.
P. J. M.

ACKNOWLEDGEMENTS

It is obvious that in producing any book, authors are dependent on a great number of people for their help and support. Indeed, if one attempted to acknowledge all those involved in this way, it would substantially lengthen the book itself. Initially, therefore, we want to record our thanks to all those who have been involved—students and staff—in helping with photographs, correcting mistakes and perhaps most of all in helping us to pitch the level of teaching at a suitable level.

The need to thank certain people specifically, however, cannot be avoided, nor would we wish to do so. The text of some 55 000 words has been typed through three phases and for the vast bulk of this we owe a great debt of thanks to Mrs G. Appleyard. To Mrs E. Pennington, who stepped into the breach at the last minute, thus enabling us to meet our copy deadline, our gratitude is also due.

The illustrations and line diagrams have all been patiently prepared by Miss R. Bailey of the Medical Illustration Section of Leeds University Medical School, and photographed (along with the other plates) by Mrs B. Smith of the Leeds Dental School Photographic Department. We are grateful to Mr I. M. Vickery and Dr G. Burton for supplying *Figs*. 3.11 and 3.12 and to Cyprane (UK) for *Fig*. 4.4.

Finally to our families and friends who have lived with us through elation and depression, 'Thank you'. It is our hope that you and our students, for whom this book is primarily written, will think it has all been worth while.

CONTENTS

1. Patient Assessment — 1
2. Pharmacology of Inhalation and Intravenous Anaesthesia — 16
3. Inhalation Anaesthesia — 38
4. Inhalation Sedation (Relative Analgesia) — 68
5. Intravenous Anaesthesia — 79
6. Oral and Intravenous Sedation (including Premedication) — 93
7. Endotracheal Anaesthesia — 107
8. Complications and Emergencies — 128
   Bibliography — 144
   Index — 145

CHAPTER 1

PATIENT ASSESSMENT

The old adage, 'Prevention is better than cure', is as appropriate to general anaesthesia as it is to any other other area of medicine or surgery. There is no doubt that a large percentage of the mishaps and accidents which occur under general anaesthesia could have been and *should* have been prevented. The nature of patient assessment is to determine, from both the surgical and anaesthetic viewpoint, the suitability of the treatment proposed for each individual.

The aim of this chapter is to alert the dental surgeon to potential problems which may occur during or after anaesthesia; it does not aim to provide an epitome of medical diagnosis nor does it suggest possible treatment plans unless they are specifically related to the anaesthetic. Such details can be found in the relevant medical and surgical textbooks, and the management of such problems is regarded primarily as the responsibility of the patient's own medical practitioner. The dental surgeon must initially assess the patient, giving consideration not only to the operative procedure but also to the type of anaesthesia, local or general. This is not necessarily a desirable state of affairs since it can be argued that it is difficult to take an objective view of the patient's well being from both angles, particularly if financial considerations have any bearing on the decisions being made. Conversely, it does have the advantage of a continuous and non-fragmented approach to treatment planning with obvious opportunities for a further opinion on potentially difficult cases.

Figure 1.1 shows a flow chart which outlines the various possibilities for treating a patient, with some of the factors which may influence a particular selection. Other permutations and combinations naturally exist or there would be little else to add to the chart, and many of the potential complications are mentioned later in this chapter. Within the sections 'Sedation' and 'General Anaesthesia' some decision also has to be made as to the location of any treatment. It is clearly necessary to assess this on the basis of all known factors including patient considerations and the availability of outpatient facilities in the dental surgery and local hospital facilities. While it may be technically possible to anaesthetize a patient with a syringe, needle and anaesthetic agent, it is the obvious duty of all practitioners to provide, at the very least, a minimum level of equipment *and* trained assistance. Consequently, the average dental practice can be adapted fairly easily to provide anaesthetic machinery, emergency equipment, suction, oxygen reserves and recovery facilities for limited periods of time and for small numbers of patients. To provide full resuscitation

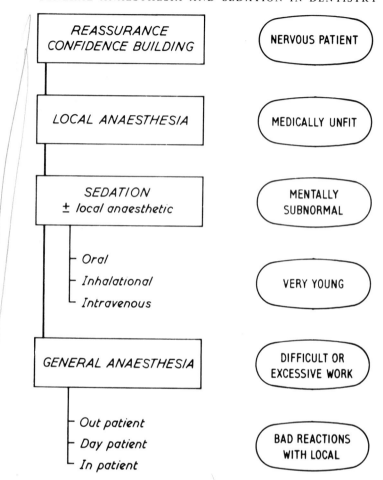

Fig. 1.1. Treatment aids and the factors influencing their use. The flow chart should be followed in principle from the top of the left-hand column taking into account the factors ringed on the right.

equipment, beds, nurses etc. is not usually practical and patients who may need such facilities should be referred to hospital.

The skill in patient evaluation comes in giving each patient informed advice as to the treatment and the type of anaesthesia that is most appropriate. The location of any recommended treatment should also be determined. Though patient assessment must obviously be carried out in the light of both medical and dental considerations, it is the former which most commonly effects limitations on the type of anaesthesia that can be used. It is impossible to produce rules on medical assessment due not only to the individual variations in patients but also because of the wide ranges of skill and experience found in both operators and anaesthetists. There are potential hazards associated with treating certain categories of patient. The more important problems are discussed in this chapter with advice on possible management; they are intended as warning lights rather than as a comprehensive guide, but the inexperienced or non-medically qualified anaesthetist would be well advised to avoid patients who do fall into these categories.

The specific considerations in the pre-anaesthetic assessment of a patient may be classified into three categories, physiological, pathological and drug-induced problems.

PHYSIOLOGICAL PROBLEMS

Age

Although age (as an isolated entity) does not pose problems, the differing metabolic rates in the very young and very old may well do. The metabolic rates of infants and young children are much higher than those of adults. Consequently, the speed at which their condition can improve or deteriorate, depending on the circumstances, can be quite remarkable. In the older person the reverse is true, since as age increases the functioning of the body system becomes progressively less efficient. While the deterioration in condition may be that much slower it is also more difficult to diagnose and may be much more profound in its effects. Careful management of all patients is essential but it should be remembered that the effects of any complication may be magnified in infants or old people. In this context it is biological age which is important and not chronological age.

Pregnancy

Pregnancy is usually considered in three 3-month periods known as trimesters. The first trimester is especially important in the formation and development of the fetus and placenta. During this sensitive period differentiation of fetal organs occurs and this may be disturbed by externally invoked stimuli. Thus all but essential drugs should be withheld from the pregnant patient and only those drugs with a proven safety record should be permitted. General anaesthetics, whether given by injection or inhalation, are drugs and clearly there can be little justification for their use, save in an emergency.

In the middle trimester there is no absolute contra-indication to general anaesthesia, because essential fetal organ development is complete and the fundus is not yet large enough to significantly affect venous return. If it is absolutely necessary to administer an anaesthetic it should be of adequate depth and, as always, the anaesthetist must ensure good oxygenation of the patient at all times.

In the final trimester it is the volume of the uterus which is the cause of most problems. It may obstruct venous return from the legs by exerting pressure on the lower part of the inferior vena cava. Reduced venous return will result in a reduced cardiac output. Anaesthetics administered in the supine position should be avoided and treatment of a faint in a pregnant woman should be to lie her head down in the lateral and not the supine position. Upward pressure of the uterine fundus may also cause delayed gastric emptying which predisposes to regurgitation of gastric contents, the inhalation of which would be life threatening. During pregnancy the maternal blood volume may be increased by up to 20% and so increased dosage of the anaesthetic agents may be necessary.

Despite the fact that pregnancy can be considered as a physiological condition it exerts profound changes on the mother's metabolism so it is considered unacceptable to anaesthetize such patients in the outpatient situation.

Psychological Difficulties

The need to determine accurately the patients' psychological and emotional states in relation to their personality cannot be emphasized too strongly. A greater percentage of patients would probably choose general anaesthesia if it were offered to them as a viable alternative to local anaesthesia, but their motives in so doing are frequently misunderstood. Even the advent of highly successful and far less painful local anaesthesia has done little to relieve the conventional attitude that dental treatment results in pain. It is for this reason, regardless of the degree of truth attached to this belief, that patients opt to have a general anaesthetic if it is offered to them. However, despite the high number of general anaesthetics given successfully every year, there can be little doubt that local anaesthesia is simpler and safer in the vast majority of patients both from the clinical and pharmacological viewpoints. In response to patient pressure it is all too easy to accede to requests for general anaesthesia rather than to try and rationalize emotional responses so that patients view treatment with less anxiety and fear. Such rationalization is preferable and of inestimable long-term benefit, since, once a patient has a tooth removed under a quick general anaesthetic, it becomes less likely that they will return to the surgery for treatment under local anaesthesia. The only beneficial alternative may be complete treatment under general anaesthesia and this is not without its difficulties. The general indications for such treatment and for administering a general anaesthetic are discussed later in this chapter.

PATIENT ASSESSMENT

PATHOLOGICAL PROBLEMS

These can be considered most conveniently by dividing the body into systems. It is advisable to remember, however, that these classifications are somewhat arbitrary and it is unusual for the effects of any one pathological condition to be limited only to the area or system it directly involves.

Cardiovascular Disorders

The cardiovascular system (CVS) is the body's primary transport system, its main function being to circulate oxygen to the tissues from the lungs, and carbon dioxide in the reverse direction. The cardiac component is regarded as a pump and the vascular component as vessels of transport and disease affecting either of these components may have serious effects during anaesthesia.

Heart disease is a common ailment in modern society and its age of onset appears to be falling. It may affect the valves, heart walls or the arteries which themselves supply the heart with the oxygen it requires. Valvular heart disease will produce a heart murmur, the significance of which can be assessed accurately by a cardiologist. Heart wall defects may also result in a murmur and again require assessment with such aids as the electrocardiogram. The effects of these diseases occupy a spectrum which extends from the asymptomatic to such problems as serious right-to-left blood shunt and/or cardiac failure. Consultation with the patient's physician is essential before deciding to proceed with any type of general anaesthesia. (It is also advisable to seek advice before administering a local anaesthetic.) Coronary artery disease can usually be diagnosed from a patient's history of chest pain, his exercise tolerance and the medications he is receiving. Its severity can be crudely estimated from the time it takes a patient to climb a flight of stairs in comfort, or the degree of pain experienced during and after exercise. Other useful pointers suggesting possible heart disease include cyanosis (a purple tinge, best observed in the fingers and lips), intermittent claudication (intermittent leg pain caused by lactic acid excesses), swelling of the ankles and venous engorgement in the jugular vein. Patients with uncomplicated angina should be advised to suck a glyceryl trinitrate tablet before treatment and should be exposed to a minimum of stress. Because of this, a safely given general anaesthetic by a competent, medically qualified anaesthetist is advisable. As an alternative, sedatives also have advantages, as they allow the surgeon to work on a conscious patient with a reduced myocardial oxygen consumption.

The vascular component of the CVS is the other factor (with the volume of blood being circulated) which affects the blood pressure in accordance with the following formula:

Blood Pressure = Cardiac Output × Peripheral Vascular Resistance.

Patients with vascular disease may present actual or potential problems during anaesthesia. Changes in blood pressure induced by anaesthetic agents, and normally tolerated in the healthy individual, may precipitate large fluctuations in the circulatory status in a patient with cardiovascular disease. This is also true for patients who are receiving corrective drug therapy. Patients with high blood pressure present an increased risk and any patient with a diastolic blood pressure over 90 mmHg should be referred for treatment. Systolic hypertension is less dangerous and is not an uncommon feature of the older patient. Large falls in blood pressure, particularly in the aged, can result in reduced cerebral and coronary perfusion with the possibility of consequent brain damage or myocardial ischaemia.

Respiratory Disorders

The respiratory system (RS) is closely related to the CVS and disease of either system can resemble features in the other. Disorders of the RS below the vocal cords are known as lower respiratory tract diseases and may include anything from a slight bronchitis in winter to an absent lung following surgical removal. Diseases above the vocal cords are known as upper respiratory tract diseases, of which infection (and particularly the common cold) is most usual. Irrespective of the pathology the problems which may occur during an anaesthetic can be of surprising proportions, particularly with diseases where excessive mucus is produced. Coughing, laryngospasm or bronchospasm can produce a frighteningly quick deterioration in the patient's well being. Despite the variation in the different conditions which may afflict the respiratory tract it is the resultant disorders of function which are important. These may be considered in relation to:

1. the amount and type of airway obstruction
2. the presence and location of secretions
3. the effect the disease has on blood gas exchange; this is affected by (1) and (2) and by the degree of compliance of the alveolar tissues of the lungs.

In patients with dental abscesses any swelling should be checked in relation to the patient's airway, in particular, when massive submandibular oedema (Ludwig's angina) is present, extreme care is needed. General anaesthetics for such patients should only be given by inhalation and under no circumstances is intravenous induction used. The importance of respiratory disorders in general anaesthesia must be emphasized since the respiratory function is vital in oxygen/carbon dioxide exchanges and in the uptake and elimination of anaesthetic gases. The physiology and pharmacology of these processes is explained in more detail in the following chapter. General anaesthesia should be postponed for patients with acute respiratory infections and patients with chronic disorders should be referred for a medical opinion. Patients suffering from debilitating respiratory disorders should be regarded as unsuitable for outpatient anaesthesia.

In recent years, however, anaesthetists have developed greater skills in understanding the management of patients suffering from respiratory disorders, and it is preferable to seek their opinion before deciding that someone is unsuitable for general anaesthesia.

Haematological Disorders

From birth to adulthood the volume of blood increases from about 300 ml to about 5 litres. About 45% of the blood is made up of cells, the majority of which are red blood cells. Their red colour is due to the presence of oxygenated haemoglobin which, when it is deoxygenated, has a blue tinge. The presence of more than 50 g/l of deoxygenated haemoglobin in the blood results in a condition known as cyanosis—a clinical term describing the colour involved and not implying any directly consequential pathology. In the healthy patient cyanosis indicates a failure of oxygen supply and should never be ignored. It should be noted that the converse is not necessarily true. Failure of the oxygen supply may not result in cyanosis in patients with anaemia due to the low quantities of haemoglobin available to be deoxygenated. The actual amount of oxygen carried in the blood depends on the quantity and nature of the haemoglobin and the degree of its oxygenation.

The quantity of haemoglobin present is dependent on a balance between its loss and replacement. Excessive loss or inadequate replacement reduce the haemoglobin content and result in an anaemia of which there are several types. Details of these are to be found in relevant medical textbooks. All anaemias affect general anaesthesia but two types of anaemia have a special significance in that general anaesthesia may aggravate the underlying disease to such an extent that it may become life threatening.

The first of these is sickle cell anaemia, an inherited disorder in which the red blood cells contain a variable amount of an abnormal haemoglobin (Hbs). It is found in under 10% of people of African and West Indian origin and far less commonly in people of Southern European origin. It occurs rarely in other races.

Sickle cell disorders are hereditary diseases with two types being recognized. The first is a homozygous form, usually called sickle cell disease, in which all the patient's haemoglobin is of the abnormal (Hbs) type. Because of its abnormal (sickle) shape it tends to be unstable and haemolyses when subjected to a reduced oxygen tension. Dehydration, stasis of the circulation and pyrexia are other factors which predispose to sickling. Severe anaemia is common and the prognosis is not good, few patients reaching the fourth decade. This group obviously presents a real anaesthetic risk and should be referred to hospital for treatment. The homozygous form of the disease is an autosomal recessive. It can, therefore, occur only in children of parents both of whom have the heterozygous form. Patients with the sickle cell trait (heterozygous form) can be assayed by means of a simple blood test to establish the amount of abnormal haemoglobin that is present. If the percentage of abnormal haemoglobin (Hbs) is low they can be fairly safely anaesthetized with an increased inspired oxygen concentration. The simple sickle cell test does not differentiate between the homozygous and heterozygous types and electrophoresis must be performed in all patients in whom a haemogloblin S solubility test is positive.

Another disease known as thalassaemia, which occurs primarily, but not solely, in mid and southern Europe, results in suppression of the production of normal haemoglobin. This can lead to a severe hypochromic anaemia which is often extremely difficult to treat. Rarely thalassaemia and sickle cell disease occur together. Such patients are at high risk during anaesthesia and must be referred to hospital for any treatment.

Other haematological disorders may affect the white blood cells or the platelets. Any problems posed are usually related to the dental work involved. Problems of prolonged bleeding or delayed healing must be borne in mind before requesting any type of anaesthesia and the treatment being given to patients for these conditions may also influence any dental procedure being planned.

The same is usually true of patients who have disorders of the blood clotting (haemostasis) system. When anaesthetics must be given they should be given by experts and injections avoided if at all possible. Haemostatic disorders may be intrinsic or extrinsic (drug induced). The intrinsic problems may be due to defects in the clotting mechanism (e.g. haemophilia) or to the initial bleeding arrest mechanism (e.g. thrombocytopoenia). Correct treatment either locally or systemically is the only way to rectify or prevent blood loss. It is salutary to remember that death results following a 30% acute loss of blood volume!

Endocrine and Metabolic Disorders

Diabetes, thyroid problems or adrenal insufficiency are endocrine disorders which pose the most problems; each of these may be secondary to a pituitary disorder.

The diabetic patient needs to be starved before anaesthesia and this is bound to upset the stability of the blood sugar levels. For this reason it is not advisable to attempt outpatient general anaesthesia. In hospital patients can be observed easily, and with modern electronic and computerized aids the blood sugar levels can be monitored precisely and controlled continuously should this be necessary.

PATIENT ASSESSMENT

Patients with thyroid disorders should be stabilized before they are anaesthetized if at all possible. There is little increased risk to a well-stabilized patient during anaesthesia, while the reverse is true of the patient suffering from either hyperthyroidism (when he may have a persistent tachycardia or atrial fibrillation) or hypothyroidism—myxoedema (when bradycardia and mental retardation may be seen). Such patients should be admitted to hospital.

Adrenal gland or pituitary gland diseases pose potentially dangerous complications. The response to stress is suppressed and there may be a secondary insulin-resistant diabetes. Oedema may be present and an increase in blood pressure may also result. Added together there is a considerable risk in anaesthetizing these patients and they should be referred for hospital treatment.

Metabolic disorders are rare but of the more common galactosaemia, phenylketonuria and maple-syrup disease are encountered from time to time. Such patients often require general anaesthesia due to their mental retardation. Hospital admission is essential, if possible under the care of their consultant physician.

Disorders of the Kidney and Liver

Amongst other functions these two organs are primarily responsible for the body's excretion processes. In particular, the kidney is responsible for the central control of the water and electrolyte balance between the blood fluids and the tissue fluids. It also plays a major role in the regulation of blood pressure. If the kidney and liver fail to balance the body requirements by excreting sufficient amounts of surplus inorganic substances the effects can be relayed to all the other body systems. The most immediate of these is the respiratory system where any acidaemia or alkalaemia will be compensated for in the respiratory centre by over or under breathing.

Further secondary disease in any of the other body systems may also follow. With disorders of the kidney the response to drugs (including anaesthetic agents) can be very variable since the rate at which they are cleared may be delayed or accelerated. The presentation of patients suffering from kidney disease is variable as is the nature of the disease itself. The appearance of good health may hide a serious problem which, with injudicious handling, could become a crisis.

The liver is a large, complex organ and is involved in the digestive, metabolic and excretory processes of the body. Impairment of liver function is a serious problem and is usually the result of infective, atrophic or neoplastic change. Occasionally damage is due to toxic drug effects and certain anaesthetic agents (particularly halothane in repeated doses) have been implicated. Liver function can be easily measured so that any patient with a suspicious history should be referred for medical opinion.

Disorders of the Nervous System

The nervous system is a complex organization of cells and fibres which receive, perceive and transmit impulses. It is particularly to the brain that the flow of oxygenated blood must be guaranteed during anaesthesia.

Certain conditions as diverse as epilepsy, spasticity, myasthenia gravis and multiple sclerosis can present problems in anaesthesia. Treatment of these diseases is often complex; in particular, patients with myasthenia gravis should be treated with immense care. Any drug which may affect muscle tone should be avoided and general anaesthetics or sedatives should only be administered in places where full emergency facilities are available. The epileptic patient should be starved for an anaesthetic and should be instructed to take his usual anti-convulsant preparations in the normal dosage. A *small* volume of water may be justifiably consumed in this action.

Other Problem Areas

In addition to the more obvious disease patterns there are several indistinct regions where assessment can prove very difficult. In these problem areas caution is advisable. They include:

1. Patients with a history of difficult anaesthesia. The information conveyed by the patient is usually sketchy and does not always appear rational. It may vary in significance from the fact that they vomited postoperatively to their being hypersensitive to suxamethonium (*see* p. 124).

Careful questioning may reveal the nature of any previous complications, but it is wise to make reference to the patient's medical practitioner (or, if possible, the anaesthetist involved) if any part of the history appears suspicious.

2. Patients who are clearly unwell. In this category it is necessary to weigh up the benefits from treatment against the problems of the anaesthetic. If the cause of the malaise is dental in origin it may be preferable to proceed with an anaesthetic and eliminate the cause. A raised temperature signifies a raised metabolic rate and this should be borne in mind. Consequently, if the treatment is not urgent it is advisable for it to be postponed until the patient is again in good health.

3. Physically handicapped or mentally handicapped patients may pose anaesthetic difficulties. Many physically handicapped patients tolerate local anaesthesia well and even moderately severe spastics can be treated with intravenous sedation if necessary. If the physical handicap is so severe that it makes local anaesthesia truly impossible the chances are that general anaesthesia may also prove difficult to administer. Adaptability and improvisation with such patients will often solve seemingly difficult problems but when possible local anaesthesia should be used. This is particularly important in patients with physical disorders of the back,

PATIENT ASSESSMENT

neck or temporomandibular joints where the airway may be compromised.

Mentally handicapped patients often require general anaesthesia for all treatment, and since they will not tolerate dentures well, conservation should be attempted whenever possible. Patients with mongolism (Down's Syndrome) are frequently overweight and have congenital heart defects. Their tongues are large and they have narrow throats with large tonsils and adenoids. In total they can present a fairly complex anaesthetic problem. The possibility of treatment using local anaesthesia should not be overlooked.

DRUG-INDUCED PROBLEMS

All drugs are intended to have an effect on one or more systems or organs of the body, and in addition can produce coincidental side-effects which may be considered either desirable or non-desirable. The nature of these reactions can be found in the relevant pharmacology textbooks and only those drugs which may affect general anaesthesia are dealt with in this section.

Drugs are for the most part beneficial and it is in the patient's interest to continue receiving them in their normal routine. The exceptions to this general rule are patients who are receiving steroid preparations of any form. In this context it should be remembered that certain skin preparations contain powerful steroids and that patients who use these liberally may require steroid cover. A physician's advice is desirable but usually a doubling of the dosage of the medication prescribed, being slowly reduced to normal over a period of 7 days will compensate for any suppression of the response to stress. Coping with a steroid crisis is dealt with in the chapter on emergencies.

The other major exception is in people who are taking anticoagulants. These present no real contra-indication to general anaesthesia but it may be necessary to reduce the dosage to allow haemostasis following surgery. If the patient is to be intubated an oral tube is both easier and safer since it reduces the risk of bleeding from the easily traumatized nasal mucosa. The oral tube may make life a little awkward for the surgeon in that it restricts access to the mouth.

Great care should be taken with patients who are on drugs for psychiatric reasons (including patients who may be drug addicts). Two types of anti-depressant—the tricyclic group of compounds and the mono-amine oxidase inhibitors (MAOI) used in the treatment of endogenous and exogenous depression respectively—can produce reactions with anaesthetic agents. The risk under general anaesthesia is greater from the MAOI, particularly when opiate derivatives are used. The tricyclic compounds tend to react with the catecholamines which are often added to local anaesthetics. In either case reaction will result in hypertensive crisis, which has occasionally resulted in mortality.

FORMING A TREATMENT PLAN

The formation of a treatment plan was outlined in the introduction to this chapter but it deserves further consideration.

Having ascertained the medical history the practitioner should be in a reasonable position to answer the question, Is this patient fit for a general anaesthesia? If he is not fit for general anaesthesia, is he fit for local anaesthesia? These questions should be answered without reference to the work intended since a patient is either fit for general anaesthesia or he is not. The duration or difficulty of a procedure is something which requires separate assessment before a viable treatment plan can be offered, but it is only a fool who will attempt a procedure under general anaesthesia on the basis of its simplicity or brevity when the patient is considered basically unfit.

On the assumption that a patient is fit for general anaesthesia it is important that there is a genuine clinical need for general anaesthesia. The fact that patients request general anaesthesia is only one of the factors to be considered in the decision and it is reasonable to complete all treatment under local anaesthesia unless:

1. It is impossible for some pathological reason, e.g. the presence of swelling or marked trismus. These conditions could also pose problems with general anaesthesia.

2. Teeth in different quadrants require extraction. Even so, removal of teeth in ipsilateral quadrants during one visit, and on the opposite side the next, make such treatment perfectly viable under local anaesthesia.

3. A patient cannot tolerate treatment with local anaesthesia, even with sedation. This should be a proven fact and not just the patient's own hypothesis. The use of oral premedication may be helpful in assessing the likely response to sedation, allowing the possibility of proceeding with either a general anaesthetic or a sedative (with local anaesthesia).

4. Patients with bleeding disorders such as haemophilia, Christmas disease or von Willebrand's disease. Those receiving anticoagulant therapy can also be included in this category. In all such patients it is important to avoid injections particularly intra-oral nerve blocks where most of the nerves concerned have small arteries and veins accompanying them.

5. Patients with a proven allergic or hypersensitive response to local anaesthetic agent. A simple faint does not qualify in this category. Where there is any doubt it is advisable to refer the patient to a dermatologist or to one of the specialist units investigating allergy to local anaesthetics found in some of the University Dental Schools.

PATIENT ASSESSMENT

6. The final factor to be considered is the attitudes of the surgeon and anaesthetist. There is little doubt that this is often a major factor in influencing a patient's choice of anaesthetic but it should be significant only after considering the patient's true interest.

The mortality from general anaesthesia is certainly low but it is much higher than that following local anaesthesia, even combined with sedation. Thus sedation can offer an attractive alternative to the patient who requests general anaesthesia solely because of anxiety and fear. Many such people not only accept and tolerate sedation but find it preferable due to the more unpleasant side-effects of general anaesthesia. Because of these advantages it is not unreasonable to pressurize patients into accepting sedation rather then general anaesthesia. If, however, having considered the patient's well being general anaesthesia is advised, the dental surgeon usually has three alternatives.

Firstly, patients with a large amount of complex work, or patients who have medical problems, can be admitted to hospital and kept 1 or 2 days before and after the operation to check that they are fit initially for the anaesthetic and operation and subsequently for discharge. Secondly, patients who are fit and well but need a slightly prolonged procedure can be admitted as day case patients in the morning and can be discharged later the same day. The third alternative is to use an 'open' general anaesthetic either in the surgery or in a hospital, when the patient should be fit and the work not too extensive. Dental outpatient general anaesthesia is unique in that the surgeon and the anaesthetist compete for control of the patient's airway. It is often the failure to co-operate in this competition and to see that protection of the patient's airway should be a common goal, which leads to accidents, some of which are fatal. Prolonged procedures which may prejudice the patient's airway should be avoided since as the operator and anaesthetist get tired the difficulties frequently increase, due to blood in the mouth, salivary flow and the possibility of teeth fracturing during extractions. Careful assessment is aimed at foreseeing these problems and preventing them.

Preparation of Patients for Anaesthesia

Patients who are to be admitted to hospital can be easily prepared for general anaesthesia but those who are to have dental outpatient general anaesthesia must be carefully instructed verbally and in writing as to their responsibilities before and after an anaesthetic. *Figure* 1.2 shows a sample set of instructions, the rationale for which is discussed below.

The patient should be starved before an anaesthetic. In general terms this means that they should have had nothing to eat or drink for at least 6 h before their appointment and only light snacks during the morning of an anaesthetic due later in the day. Long periods of starvation are inadvisable since the build-up of acidic gastric juices can heighten the

> **GENERAL ANAESTHETIC INSTRUCTIONS**
> *If you do not follow these instructions your appointment will be cancelled*
>
> # YOU MUST:
>
> 1. NOT eat or drink anything for six hours before your appointment
> 2. Come with a responsible adult who can take you home
> 3. NOT drive or operate any type of machinery, or drink alcoholic beverages for 24 hours after your operation
> 4. Inform the anaesthetist if you take any medicine on prescription
> 5. Inform the anaesthetist if and when you last had an anaesthetic
>
> YOUR APPOINTMENT IS AT...................ON.................................
>
> ORAL SURGERY SERVICES (LEEDS)

Fig. 1.2. A sample appointment card giving the important pre-anaesthetic instructions.

vomiting reflex. If these are vomited and inhaled during an anaesthetic they are more dangerous than aqueous drinks. Some of the inflexible rules regarding starving patients are not always logical and whilst it is not permissible to have eaten within 6 h of an anaesthetic, small quantities of aqueous fluids (not milk or alcohol) may be consumed up to 4 h before the appointment.

Escorts should be responsible adults who can bring the patient to and from the surgery. Wherever possible this should be in a taxi or private car. Public transport is acceptable but riding pillion passenger on a motor cycle is not. Patients should be warned against driving, operating machinery or drinking alcoholic drinks for a period of 24 h following the administration of a general anaesthetic or sedative.

A few minutes before the anaesthetic they should be instructed to visit the lavatory as control of the bladder under general anaesthesia is extremely variable.

All dentures, appliances, glasses, contact lenses, loose jewellery and watches should be removed. It is also advisable to remove lipstick and nail varnish (so that the lips and fingernails can be monitored for cyanosis) and mascara (which can irritate the eyes). The above instructions should be given in writing and reinforced verbally.

PATIENT ASSESSMENT

Written consent in which patients sign that they agree to the type of anaesthetic, the planned procedure and any necessary alternatives should be obtained from patients who are over sixteen. The parents or guardians of children below sixteen should sign on their behalf.

The patient can then be taken to the surgery where the anaesthetic is to be given. The anaesthetist should check that the patient has complied with the instructions that were given and the medical history should be rechecked. Although this adds time it is a valuable safeguard. It should be done systematically and without asking leading questions such as 'You haven't had breakfast, have you?' It is far more reliable to ask when patients last had anything to eat or drink. The patient should be asked to loosen any tight clothing which may reduce their inspiratory capabilities. The patency of the nasal airways is then checked blocking each nostril in turn and asking the patient to inhale deeply.

The dental surgeon should finally recheck the treatment plan, particularly that he and the anaesthetist are happy that the treatment proposed is not excessive for the type of anaesthetic about to be administered.

The mouth should be checked for loose crowns or loose teeth and the anaesthetist warned accordingly. It is often suggested that any painful teeth are identified so they can be removed first in case the anaesthetic has to be abandoned before treatment is complete.

If all is in order the dental surgeon can stand aside and the anaesthetist can proceed.

CHAPTER 2

PHARMACOLOGY OF INHALATION AND INTRAVENOUS ANAESTHESIA

The safe practical use of all anaesthetic agents requires an understanding of their pharmacology. All too often the acquisition of pharmacological fact is seen as the key to a particular undergraduate or postgraduate examination when in reality, it forms, with physiology, the basis of safe clinical practice. Before discussing the properties of the individual agents in the latter half of the chapter, it is important to out-line the general physiology and pharmacology as it applies to anaesthesia in general. A short section on the role of oxygen is also included as it is of fundamental importance.

INHALATIONAL ANAESTHESIA

All general anaesthetic agents produce anaesthesia by their action on various areas in the brain. The degree of their activity, i.e. the depth of anaesthesia, is proportional to their partial pressure at the site of action. This may be thought of as the force with which the dissolved gas is attempting to come out of solution. Inhalational anaesthetics reach the brain by entering the lungs, crossing the alveolar membranes into the blood, returning with the blood to the left side of the heart and thence in the arterial blood to the tissues of the body. Thus the two main aspects of inhalational anaesthesia are entry of the agent with the inspired anaesthetic gases into the lungs and distribution of the agent, by the circulation, to the tissues.

Entry into the Lungs

The inhalational anaesthetic agents in current use are administered as gases or vapours. Gases are stored in a compressed form in steel cylinders. Within the cylinder they may be gaseous (e.g. oxygen) or liquid (nitrous oxide). In either case they emerge from the cylinder as gases and their flow rates are controlled by needle valves via calibrated rotameters. Vapours are dispensed from some form of calibrated vaporizer. Since the liquid has to be vaporized the calibration is usually expressed as a percentage, and the primary gases are mixed with it. The inspired mixture of gases is then administered by way of an appropriate anaesthetic circuit. Accurate control over the composition of the inspired agents is essential, not only to allow control of the depth of anaesthesia, but also to ensure that the patient inspires a mixture of gases containing sufficient oxygen to maintain the partial pressure of oxygen in the arterial blood at an adequate level (*see* p. 29).

By virtue of their mode of administration via the lungs, the inhalational agents are dependent upon respiration for their entry into the body and some understanding of the respiratory system is essential. Respiration is controlled by groups of neurones in the brain stem collectively referred to as the respiratory centre. This centre receives sensory information from various groups of receptors situated in the brain, the major blood vessels, the lungs and the respiratory muscles. Chemoreceptors, sensitive to the hydrogen ion activity (pH) in the cerebrospinal fluid (CSF), on the surface of the medulla convey chemical information concerning the partial pressure of carbon dioxide (Pa_{CO_2}) in the blood. Any acute rise or fall in the Pa_{CO_2} will be quickly accompanied by a change in the pH in the environment of the chemoreceptors, as carbon dioxide is soluble and quickly diffuses across the blood-brain barrier into the CSF. CSF has a relatively poor buffering capacity and the extra hydrogen ions produced by the carbon dioxide in solution forming carbonic acid will rapidly alter the CSF pH.

$$CO_2 + H_2O \rightleftharpoons H_2CO_3 \rightleftharpoons H^+ + HCO_3^-$$

The respiratory response to changes in Pa_{CO_2} is very strong indeed in normal individuals, a rise in Pa_{CO_2} of 1 mmHg causing an increase in ventilation of about 2·5 litres/min.

This sensitivity of the brain stem chemoreceptors can be reduced by chronic exposure to an increased Pa_{CO_2} such as would be caused by chronic bronchitis.

Chemoreceptors in the carotid bodies, which have a very generous blood supply, have a very high oxygen consumption and respond to falls in the partial pressure of oxygen (Pa_{O_2}) in the arterial blood. However, in contrast to the response to carbon dioxide relatively large changes in Pa_{O_2} are required to produce hyperventilation and significant changes in ventilation are only seen when the Pa_{O_2} has fallen by 50%.

Stretch receptors are present in the lungs and respiratory muscles, and convey information to the respiratory centre about the state of inflation of the lungs, and the compliance of the chest wall. This information is used by the respiratory centre to provide breath by breath control over the depth of respiration. Important tactile receptors and chemoreceptors are present in the mucosa of the upper and lower respiratory tract and are responsible for initiating such complex mechanisms as coughing, sneezing and bronchiolar constriction in response to noxious stimuli.

Higher brain centres associated with the emotions (e.g. fear or excitement) and/or voluntary influences can alter the pattern of respiration, as can other sensory modalities outside the respiratory system (e.g. pain).

The respiratory centre drives the muscles of respiration via the spinal cord and the peripheral nerves. All the commonly used inhalational, intravenous and local anaesthetic agents can influence this control of respiration by acting at several points along the control system outlined in *Fig.* 2.1. The nature of the interference will be discussed when considering

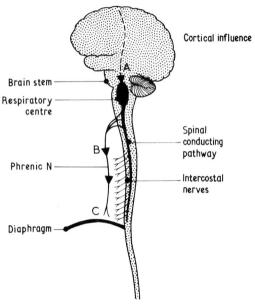

Fig. 2.1. Influences on the control of respiration. At site A, the respiratory centre is depressed by all the modern, potent inhalation agents, the narcotic analgesics and the intravenous induction agents. At site B, the phrenic nerve is only affected by regional nerve block using local anaesthetic. At site C, the neuromuscular junction is influenced by the neuromuscular blocking agents and to a lesser extent by halothane and enflurane.

each individual agent. The phrenic nerve initiates activity in the diaphragm which is the major muscle driving the spontaneous ventilation of the lungs. However, various accessory muscles of respiration become involved during circumstances requiring increased respiratory activity such as exercise or in airway obstruction. The activity of these accessory muscles is a valuable sign during anaesthesia that the patient is being forced to employ extra effort to achieve adequate ventilation. Since it is the respiratory centre which monitors the effects of ventilatory activity on clearance of carbon dioxide and uptake of oxygen by the lungs, it is clear that for increased activity to be instituted by the respiratory centre a change for the worse must have occurred in the blood reaching the brain.

Contraction of the diaphragm, in conjuction with the action of the intercostal muscles, pulling the ribs upwards and outwards increases the volume of the thoracic cavity and creates a sub-atmospheric pressure (*not* a negative pressure) in the chest. In response to the increased pressure gradient thus created air rushes in through the mouth and nose, and via the pharynx, larynx, trachea and bronchi to the respiratory bronchioles and alveoli. Here, by crossing the alveolar membrane, oxygen diffuses into the blood. This whole process is called inspiration. During expiration the muscles of respiration relax, the thorax and diaphragm return to their original dimensions and the alveolar air, carrying with it carbon dioxide, is expelled. This continuing sequence of inspiration and expiration is essential for the induction, maintenance and recovery from an inhaled general anaesthetic.

The volume of air involved in each breath is called the tidal volume and is typically about 450 ml at rest in a 70-kg adult. Combined with a respiratory frequency of some 12 breaths/min, this results in a volume of about 5 litres/min, the so-called 'minute volume'. This can be represented by the formula:

$$\text{Minute volume} = \text{Tidal volume} \times \text{Respiratory rate}$$

Of the 450 ml air taken in during inspiration only two-thirds (about 300 ml) reaches the alveoli to take part in gaseous exchange with the blood. The remaining one-third (or 150 ml) of each breath is called the dead space as it occupies the volume of the conducting airways, i.e. nose, pharynx, larynx, trachea, bronchi and bronchioles, in which no significant gaseous exchange takes place. Dead space can be significantly increased by poorly designed anaesthetic apparatus (which will reduce the efficiency of gaseous exchange) and by disease processes in the patient, e.g. chronic bronchitis.

During the induction of inhalational anaesthesia each breath of anaesthetic mixture incrementally raises the partial pressure of anaesthetic in the alveoli. Some of this anaesthetic then diffuses across the alveolar membrane into the blood. The solubility in blood of the specific agent being used is crucial in determining how quickly its partial pressure in the alveoli, and thus the blood and the brain, will rise. A rapid rate of rise of partial pressure means a rapid onset of effect during induction and a rapid clearance of the agent during recovery. These rates are largely dependent on the solubility of the agents. Solubility in blood is expressed as the 'blood gas distribution coefficient'.* For a soluble agent, e.g. diethyl ether, with a blood gas distribution coefficient of approximately 13, the blood will be able to dissolve or take up a large quantity of the agent at a low partial pressure. The consequence of this is that large amounts of this agent will have to be administered in order to produce an effective rise in the partial pressure in the tissues and therefore induction of anaesthesia

---

* Blood gas distribution (partition) coefficient is the ratio of the number of molecules of the agent in the blood phase to the number of molecules in the gaseous phase per unit volume at equilibrium.

will be slow. In general terms, therefore, partial pressure is inversely proportional to the solubility.

Ultimately it is the inspired concentration of the anaesthetic agent (i.e. the amount being administered to the patient from the vaporizer/flow meter) that will finally determine the depth of anaesthesia. Higher inspired concentrations will also tend to increase the speed of induction of anaesthesia as more anaesthetic will reach the alveoli with each breath. However, the irritant effects of higher concentrations may prevent the patient breathing the agent and the agent itself may depress respiration, both of these effects limiting the uptake of anaesthetic.

Two other factors are of great importance in determining the rapidity of onset of anaesthesia. It is clear that any increases in minute volume, such as can be caused by telling the patient to take deep breaths, will also increase the delivery of anaesthetic to the lungs. Unfortunately this will also clear more carbon dioxide from the blood with a resultant reduced respiratory drive from the respiratory centre. This, coupled with the respiratory depression of which most of the potent inhalational agents are capable, will once again slow the uptake of anaesthetic. The reduction in blood carbon dioxide tension will itself decrease the cerebral blood flow which again will reduce the delivery of anaesthetic to the brain.

The remaining important factor is the cardiac output, i.e. the blood flowing through the lungs. The cardiac output is the volume of blood ejected per minute by the left ventricle into the systemic circulation and is expressed in litres per minute. It is this volume of blood which, in its passage through the lungs, takes up the anaesthetic agent and carries it to the tissues of the body. If the cardiac output is high then a relatively large volume of blood will be passing through the lungs per minute. Thus the anaesthetic agent present in the lungs will be taken up into this larger volume of blood, and since concentration = mass per unit volume the concentration of anaesthetic in the blood will be low. Conversely, in situations where the cardiac output is low the anaesthetic available in the lungs will be taken up by a smaller volume of blood and therefore its concentration in the blood will be higher.

The clinical importance of this will be that a high cardiac output will result in a slower rise in partial pressure of anaesthetic in the blood and hence a slower induction of anaesthesia. This merely reinforces the intuitive feeling, supported by practical experience, that a calm relaxed patient can be anaesthetized more quickly and smoothly than an excited agitated one.

One further factor must be briefly mentioned, that of the 'second gas effect'. When the inhalation of an anaesthetic mixture containing at least two component gases is commenced (e.g. nitrous oxide, oxygen and halothane) and where one component (in this case nitrous oxide) is present in moderately high concentration (70%), the initial rapid uptake of the nitrous oxide by the blood will result in an increased uptake of the other agents. The basis for the increased uptake of the second agent has two possible causes. Firstly, large volumes of nitrous oxide are taken up by the blood from the alveoli and further anaesthetic mixture moves into the space thus created. Secondly, Dalton's law of partial pressures states that the ambient pressure in the alveoli is the sum of the partial pressures of the component gases. If the partial pressure of one of the component gases is reduced by uptake, then there will be a relative increase in the partial pressure of the other agents.

Anaesthetic Potency

The term potency when applied to inhaled anaesthetics has three possible interpretations.

1. The speed of onset of action of the agent, i.e. potency, is synonymous with blood gas distribution coefficient or solubility.
2. The depth of anaesthesia attainable with the agent in terms of narcosis and muscle relaxation.
3. The concentration of the agent required to abolish the response to a standard surgical stimulus.

Of these three the last is currently taken as the definition of potency, and the potency is now expressed in terms of a minimal alveolar concentration (MAC) value for the agent. The MAC of the agent is that inspired concentration of the agent which will, at equilibrium, abolish the response to a standard surgical stimulus in 50% of patients. Although the inspired concentration is measured as a percentage, MAC is usually expressed merely as a number. The term 'at equilibrium' indicates the condition in which the tissue concentration is equal to the inspired concentration and depending upon the solubility of the agent may take many hours to achieve. An important feature of MAC values is that they are additive, i.e. 0·5 MAC of nitrous oxide plus 0·5 MAC halothane equals 1 MAC of anaesthesia. MAC is a useful index of anaesthetic potency which has its basis in clinical practice, i.e. the response to a surgical stimulus, and it also correlates reasonably well with previous standards of potency such as lipid solubility which is an expression of the oil–gas distribution coefficient.

INDIVIDUAL ANAESTHETIC AGENTS

The inhalation anaesthetic agents in widespread use in the UK today are nitrous oxide, halothane and enflurane. No doubt trichloroethylene and possibly even ether are still used by those practitioners unwilling to give up agents with which they are familiar and which have proved reliable in long use. However, it is unlikely that students in training today will see either trichloroethylene or ether in use. Hopefully the use of ethyl chloride and chloroform has long been abandoned, as both agents are associated with episodes of cardiac arrest in situations where the patient has high endogenous catecholamine levels. The explosive agent cyclopropane, still used occasionally for gaseous induction for children, is also virtually obsolete.

Accordingly, nitrous oxide, halothane, enflurane and isoflurane are discussed and a section on oxygen uptake and transport is included as it is fundamentally associated with inhalational techniques. For historical interest a few lines are included on agents such as ether, trichloroethylene, ethyl chloride and chloroform, although these agents have been superseded.

Nitrous Oxide

Nitrous oxide (N_2O) was discovered in 1776 by Joseph Priestley, who was well aware of the effects produced by this agent, describing the sensation as 'an highly pleasurable thrilling, particularly in the chest and extremities'. In 1799 another famous scientist, Humphry Davy, observed the analgesic properties of nitrous oxide and actually proposed its use in surgical operation, a suggestion which passed unheeded. It fell to a dental surgeon, Mr Horace Wells of Hartford, Connecticut, USA, to introduce nitrous oxide as an anaesthetic agent in December 1844. At that time public demonstrations of nitrous oxide inhalation were given at county fairs by travelling 'lecturers in chemistry' and it was at such a demonstration given by one Quincy Coulton, that Wells rediscovered the previously noted analgesic properties of nitrous oxide and decided to put them to use in his own dental practice. In thoroughly commendable spirit he himself was the first patient, prior to using the technique on his patients.

Nitrous oxide is a colourless non-irritant inorganic gas with a faintly sweet smell, of molecular weight 44·0 daltons and at a specific gravity of 1·53 (air = 1·0) which liquefies at $-89\,°C$ at atmospheric pressure. It is manufactured by heating ammonium nitrate to between 250 and 270 °C and the resulting nitrous oxide is purified and compressed into cylinders at 50 atmospheres pressure (505 kPa).

$$NH_4NO_3 \longrightarrow N_2O + 2H_2O$$

Ammonia, nitric acid and the higher oxides of nitrogen, nitric oxide (NO) and nitrogen dioxide (NO_2) are all possible contaminants of the gas and great efforts are made to remove them, particularly the higher oxides of nitrogen, as a death has occurred in clinical practice due to contamination of nitrous oxide with NO/NO_2.

The nitrous oxide is easily compressed into liquid form at a pressure of approximately 505 kPa and is sold by weight in blue cylinders, each cylinder being stamped with its empty weight. As the contents of the cylinder are liquid the pressure inside the cylinder, as measured on the pressure gauge of the anaesthetic machine, will reflect the saturated vapour pressure of that liquid, i.e. nitrous oxide, at the temperature of measurements. The saturated vapour pressure of a liquid only varies with temperature, thus one might expect the pressure inside the cylinder to remain constant during use until all the liquid had evaporated. However, in order to evaporate a liquid, heat is required and the latent heat of vaporization (i.e. the heat required to change the substance from the liquid phase to the gaseous or vapour phase) is obtained from the metal cylinder and the surrounding atmosphere. The consequent drop in temperature results in a fall in the saturated vapour pressure within the cylinder and the observed pressure therefore falls as the temperature falls. Should the flow from the cylinder be turned off, the observed pressure in the cylinder will rise as the temperature of the cylinder slowly returns to room temperature. Should any liquid nitrous oxide still remain in the cylinder the pressure seen on the machine gauge will once again appear to indicate a full cylinder, despite the fact that it may be almost empty. With continuous use frost is frequently seen on the outside of the cylinder, and the temperature can fall low enough to sufficiently reduce the saturated vapour pressure so that the pressure in the cylinder fails to open the reducing valves on some anaesthetic machines.

Nitrous oxide is a weak anaesthetic with an MAC value greater than 100, i.e. surgical anaesthesia with adequate oxygenation cannot usually be achieved at atmospheric pressure by this agent alone. Its former use as the sole inhaled gas, i.e. 100% nitrous oxide inhalation for the induction of anaesthesia or the extraction of teeth, is a dangerous practice not to be contemplated. It is a potent analgesic which at 50% inhaled concentration has been equated to that of parenteral morphine injection in standard dose.

Nitrous oxide has a low blood gas partition coefficient of 0·47, i.e. it is relatively insoluble and thus its partial pressure in the blood and tissues rises rapidly and its onset of action is rapid. At saturation 45 ml gas will dissolve in 100 ml blood. A further consequence of the insolubility of this agent is that when the inhalation is discontinued the nitrous oxide dissolved in the blood is rapidly eliminated via the lungs. During the first few minutes of this elimination large volumes of nitrous oxide pour out of the blood into the lungs and can actually displace oxygen from the lungs causing the well-recognized entity of diffusion hypoxia. For this reason it is wise to give the patient supplemental oxygen via a face mask at the end of a nitrous oxide anaesthetic. It is a non-flammable and non-explosive agent which will, however, support an existing combustion since at above 450 °C the following reaction occurs

$$2N_2O \longrightarrow 2N_2 + O_2$$

producing a 33% oxygen-rich mixture.

In the body nitrous oxide is relatively inert and is not metabolized.

Physiologically it has minor cardiovascular depressant properties and its euphoriant actions on the central nervous system (causing exhilaration and hilarity) earned it the original epithet of 'laughing gas'.

Clinically it is the most widely used inhalational agent in British anaesthesia as with an appropriate inspired oxygen concentration it provides an excellent carrier vehicle for the more potent inhaled anaesthetic vapours and its rapid onset and analgesic action provide a valuable adjunct to other forms of anaesthesia.

Halothane

Halothane was first synthesized and used clinically in 1956. The result of modern organic chemical and pharmacological science, its history is understandably less romantic than that of nitrous oxide.

Halothane is a clear colourless liquid with a specific gravity of 1·7 and a characteristic smell. Thymol 0·01% is added as a stabilizer. Halothane boils at 50·2 °C at atmospheric pressure and the formula is

$$\begin{array}{c} F Br \\ | | \\ F-C-C-H \\ | | \\ F Cl \end{array}$$

It decomposes in light to form irritant acids and is therefore stored in dark glass bottles. Halothane is moderately volatile, the vapour being non-inflammable and non-explosive. The saturated vapour pressure at 20 °C is 241 mmHg (32·1 kPa) which is an important fact since it would be possible to achieve an inspired concentration of about 30% should liquid halothane spill into the anaesthetic circuit. Such an inspired concentration would rapidly prove fatal due to myocardial and respiratory depression. This emphasizes the need to administer halothane from an appropriately calibrated vaporizer which delivers a known concentration. Such a vaporizer can be as simple as the Goldman vaporizer (*see* p. 64), which is essentially a small glass container with an adjustable sleeve valve, or as complex as a Dräger vaporizer with its massive copper construction, built-in thermometers and accurate cone valve.

Halothane is a potent anaesthetic with a MAC value of 0·76. Its non-irritant properties and its moderate solubility allow satisfactory inhalation induction of anaesthesia, particularly in conjuction with a nitrous oxide–oxygen mixture. It has a blood gas coefficient of 2·4, i.e. it is moderately soluble.

The actions of halothane on the heart are clinically important. Primarily, halothane is a potent cardiac depressant causing falls in the cardiac contractile force, the heart rate and the blood pressure. These changes are dose dependent; the deeper the halothane anaesthesia, the greater the falls in cardiac output and blood pressure. Disorders of cardiac rhythm are also common during halothane anaesthesia and are related to increases in the amounts of adrenaline and noradrenaline secreted by the body. This increase in endogenous catecholamine secretion is caused both by the surgical stimulation and by the increase in Pa_{CO_2} during halothane anaesthesia.

It is for this reason that injected adrenaline must be strictly limited during halothane anaesthesia to a total dose of 10 ml of 1 : 100 000 adrenaline in any one 10-min period. The fall in blood pressure seen during halothane anaesthesia is also associated with a fall in coronary artery blood flow. However, the oxygen requirements of the myocardium are also reduced in step with this fall in blood flow and therefore halothane anaesthesia is not absolutely contra-indicated in patients with heart disease.

The increase in Pa_{CO_2} seen during halothane anaesthesia is brought about by its depressant action on the respiratory centre. The respiratory rate is usually maintained, but there is a fall in tidal volume. Typically Pa_{CO_2} values rise as high as 60 mmHg (8 kPa). This rise is relevant to the patient's oxygenation since, due to Dalton's law of partial pressures, the ambient pressure of a system (i.e. the patient's lungs) is the sum of the partial pressures contributed by the constituent gases. Thus, if the partial pressure of carbon dioxide rises then the partial pressure of the other constituent gases, usually nitrous oxide and oxygen, must fall in order for the sum of the partial pressures to remain the same. Thus, in a patient breathing spontaneously during a halothane anaesthetic the inspired oxygen concentration should be maintained at a minimum of 30%.

Bronchiolar muscle tone is also reduced by halothane. This results in an increase in the diameter of the bronchioles and a corresponding fall in airways resistance. This is of little significance in ordinary patients, but can be of great benefit in patients prone to bronchoconstriction (e.g. asthmatics).

Other important actions of halothane must be mentioned. It increases the cerebral blood flow even if the Pa_{CO_2} is rendered normal by artificial ventilation of the patient. It also causes moderate reduction in renal and hepatic blood flows. The role of halothane as an hepatotoxic agent has been raised increasingly in the last decade. To put this concern into perspective, post-halothane hepatic dysfunction following a single halothane anaesthetic is extremely rare. However, this is not the case with repeated halothane anaesthetics and although there are no concrete guidelines, it is advisable to allow a minimum period of 12 weeks to elapse before administering a repeat halothane anaesthetic. Halothane is metabolized in the liver and it is possible that the metabolites are responsible for hepatic dysfunction.

One further clinically important point to be noted is that halothane can be associated with postoperative shivering and the muscle activity so generated will cause an increased demand for oxygen. Most patients who are fit and well will be able to generate the increased cardiac output to meet this oxygen requirement. However, diffusion hypoxia (*see* p. 23) in association with shivering will produce marked hypoxaemia and supplemental oxygen should be given.

In spite of these minor drawbacks halothane has proved to be an effective, safe and reliable agent in clinical use with a predictable and controllable degree of respiratory and cardiovascular depression which is clinically acceptable.

Enflurane

Enflurane is a modern halogenated ether synthesized in 1963 and first used clinically, in 1966, in North America, where its use is now widespread. It is another clear colourless volatile liquid boiling at 56·5 °C and with its own distinctive, almost unpleasant, odour. No stabilizing agent is added and the formula is:

$$\begin{array}{c} FFF \\ ||| \\ H-C-C-O-C-H \\ ||| \\ ClFF \end{array}$$

The saturated vapour pressure is 175 mmHg (23·3 kPa) at 20 °C and it is administered from a calibrated temperature-compensated vaporizer. Enflurane is a moderately potent agent with an MAC value of 1·68 and is less soluble than halothane having a blood gas distribution coefficient of 1·91. Thus clinically one might expect to see a more rapid uptake of the agent and a quicker onset of action. In comparison with halothane the myocardial depression seen with enflurane is, if anything, greater. The falls of blood pressure seen under enflurane anaesthesia are greater than those with comparable halothane anaesthesia. However, the incidence of spontaneous cardiac arrhythmias is lower with enflurane and the use of adrenaline as a vasoconstrictor in local anaesthetic drugs is not associated with problems of cardiac rhythm.

Although it is described as a non-irritant drug the use of enflurane is associated with upper respiratory tract irritation as evidenced by an increased incidence of laryngospasm and coughing. It is also a potent respiratory depressant possibly more potent than halothane so the use of adequate inspired oxygen concentrations is, as always, mandatory.

Several other features of its use require comment. Being an ether, there is a marked degree of voluntary muscle relaxation with enflurane. This is more pronounced than with any other inhalational agent except diethyl ether itself, and there is marked potentiation of the non-depolarizing muscle relaxants. (The different types of muscle relaxant are discussed more fully in Chapter 7.) This potentiation is not regarded as being a great advantage in the UK where full paralysing doses of neuromuscular blocking agents such as curare have always been used. However, the technique of combining the actions of enflurane and the non-depolarizing relaxants has found widespread use in North America. Clinically the moderate muscle relaxation obtained with enflurane alone is useful but limited by its respiratory depressant action.

Deep anaesthesia is associated with abnormalities of the electrical activity of the brain, in which the electro-encephalogram shows high amplitude spikes and wave features reminiscent of some forms of seizure activity, which is aggravated by hypocapnoea (low Pa_{CO_2}). Thus mechanical ventilation using deep enflurane anaesthesia is most likely to induce this electrical phenomenon and is therefore contra-indicated.

Inhalational agents containing several fluorine atoms are metabolized in the liver to release free inorganic fluoride ions. Not only does the number of fluorine atoms present in the original anaesthetic molecule influence the level of the free fluoride ion seen, but also the structure of the molecule. Free fluoride levels greater than 50 mmol/l are associated with a high output renal failure. Enflurane, the molecule of which contains five fluorine atoms, is relatively innocuous being associated with a free fluoride level of only 15 mmol/l. No cases of hepatic damage have been reported following enflurane administration.

Isoflurane

Isoflurane is even more modern, being another halogenated ether of North American origin. It is an isomer of enflurane, and was isolated in 1965 and first used in human volunteers in 1971. Isoflurane is also clear and colourless, boiling at 58·5 °C. It is rather more volatile than enflurane, with a saturated vapour pressure of 33·3 kPa. The formula is:

$$F-\underset{\underset{F}{|}}{\overset{\overset{F}{|}}{C}}-\underset{\underset{Cl}{|}}{\overset{\overset{H}{|}}{C}}-O-\underset{\underset{F}{|}}{\overset{\overset{F}{|}}{C}}-H$$

It is stable with no added preservative.

Currently isoflurane is not in general use in the UK and therefore no personal experience of its pharmacological properties by the authors in patients is available. It is a potent agent (MAC 1·3) and its blood gas distribution coefficient is 1·4. These two factors would indicate that this agent might prove very useful as it is less soluble than either halothane or enflurane, and has an MAC value indicating a potency almost as great as halothane. Its action on the cardiovascular system appears to be rather different to that of the other potent inhalational agents in that cardiac output appears to be maintained, but the blood pressure falls to levels comparable with halothane and enflurane due to a fall in the systemic vascular resistance. Respiratory depression with isoflurane is also similar to that seen with the potent inhalational agents. Renal toxicity due to the fluoride ion has not been reported.

The clinical importance of these two new agents must be examined critically. At the time of writing isoflurane is not widely available in the UK but it possesses attributes likely to be useful in dental anaesthesia, namely it is potent and has a low blood gas solubility which promises a rapid induction and recovery from anaesthesia. It is, however, a difficult isomer to isolate and its cost is therefore likely to be prohibitive when and if it becomes generally available.

Enflurane is available and its lower solubility than halothane would appear to give it some advantage in terms of a more rapid induction and recovery. It also possesses the beneficial quality of apparently causing no hepatic dysfunction even with repeated use. However, its higher MAC and its high cost will probably discourage its widespread use in dental anaesthesia. It is, however, proving a useful agent in situations where repeated inhalational anaesthetics must be given.

Other Inhalational Agents

The remaining inhalational agents which have been used in the past, namely diethyl ether, trichloroethylene, chloroform and ethyl chloride, have now virtually disappeared from the anaesthetic scene.

Diethyl ether was first synthesized in 1540 by Valerius Cordus and was probably first used for anaesthesia by Crawford Long in 1842 at Jefferson, Georgia, USA. Ether has a high blood gas partition coefficient (approximately 13) and therefore the induction with ether was extremely slow with much struggling and excitement on the patient's part (*see* Chapter 3). It is a very safe agent to use as it stimulates respiration and the blood pressure and cardiac output are well maintained due to endogenous catecholamine secretion stimulated by the ether itself. A high incidence of postoperative vomiting was a further cause of its abandonment, as was its explosive nature when mixed with oxygen.

Trichloroethylene was synthesized in 1864 by Emil Fischer, and was used initially as a dry cleaning fluid. Its potent analgesic properties were recognized at the turn of the century when it was used to relieve trigeminal neuralgia. It also has a high blood gas distribution coefficient giving a slow induction and recovery. It can cause toxic damage to the cranial nerves.

The anaesthetic properties of chloroform were discovered in 1847 by Flowers, and Simpson in Edinburgh soon put it to clinical use. It allowed a more rapid, pleasant induction and recovery than did ether and it achieved widespread popularity in the UK following its administration to Queen Victoria in 1853 for the birth of Prince Leopold. The incidence of sudden death due to cardiac arrest during induction of anaesthesia with chloroform and the postoperative hepatotoxicity of this agent led to its use being abandoned.

Ethyl chloride, a highly volatile liquid, was first described as an anaesthetic in 1847. Its propensity for causing sudden cardiac arrest is similar to that of chloroform, and it too has now been abandoned.

OXYGEN UPTAKE AND TRANSPORT

Oxygen is of fundamental importance to tissue respiration in man, as the producton of adenosine triphosphate (ATP) required to drive the metabolic processes of the cells is many times more efficient during aerobic metabolism than with anaerobic metabolism. Anaerobic metabolism, i.e. cellular metabolism in the absence of oxygen, can only meet the cell's metabolic requirement for a very short time. Thus maintenance of tissue oxygenation should be the first objective during every anaesthetic.

Oxygen is present in the atmosphere constituting one-fifth or 20·93% of the volume of the air. Assuming the barometric pressure to be 1 atm, i.e. 760 mmHg (101 kPa) the partial pressure of oxygen will be 20·93% of 760, i.e. 159 mmHg (21·1 kPa). This is the partial pressure of oxygen that enters the nose and mouth during inspiration. However, the situation in the lungs is rather different. The air of the lungs taking part in gas exchange in the alveoli (the alveolar air) is a mixture of nitrogen, oxygen, carbon dioxide and water vapour. The average pressure in the lungs is virtually atmospheric, so applying Dalton's law of partial pressures (see p. 21) the partial pressure of oxygen in the alveoli must be lower than that in the inspired air.

During its passage through the upper respiratory tract the inspired air is humidified and on reaching the alveoli the air is saturated with water vapour. The saturated vapour pressure of water at 37 °C is 47 mmHg (6·2 kPa), therefore the partial pressure of oxygen in the inspired air in the lower respiratory tract is 20·93% of (760−47) which is 149 mmHg (19·8 kPa). On entering the alveoli the presence of carbon dioxide which has diffused out of the blood and across the alveolar membrane, causes a further reduction in the partial pressure of oxygen in the alveolar air to a value of approximately 100–110 mmHg (c.14 kPa). It is this level of partial pressure of oxygen in the alveoli, the PaO_2, which drives the oxygen across the alveolar membrane into the blood. The molecules of oxygen are not magically sucked into the blood, but must move down a pressure gradient. The venous blood arriving at the lungs in the pulmonary artery from the right side of the heart has a partial pressure of oxygen of about 40 mmHg (5·3 kPa) and when this blood, having traversed the pulmonary capillaries in contact with the alveoli, has picked up oxygen, its PaO_2 increases to about 95–100 mmHg (13 kPa). This is part of the process of arterializing the venous blood.

The relationship between PaO_2 and haemoglobin saturation is seen in the oxygen/haemoglobin dissociation curve, which in normal individuals shows a sigmoid shape (*Fig.* 2.2). The normal arterial point is marked at A and it can be seen that along the flat upper section of the curve from A to B, which represents the range of Pa_{O_2} commonly found in healthy adults, the haemoglobin remains more than 85% saturated with oxygen, providing the Pa_{O_2} is at least 60 mmHg (8 kPa). The part of the curve down to point C plots the change in saturation of the haemoglobin during the normal desaturation accompanying oxygen distribution to the tissues.

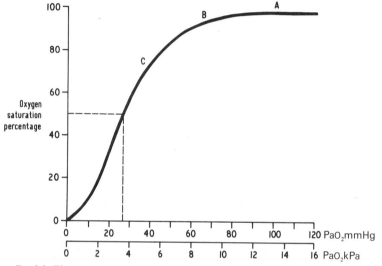

Fig. 2.2. The oxygen/haemoglobin dissociation curve.

The position of the curve can be shifted either to the right or to the left by physiological and/or physical changes.

The most common influences on the position of the curve are shown diagrammatically by the arrows in *Fig.* 2.3. A shift to the left results in an increase in the affinity of the haemoglobin for oxygen. This means that the tissue partial pressure of oxygen must fall to a lower value before oxygen will be released from the haemoglobin. Conversely, a shift in the curve to the right causes the haemoglobin to give up its oxygen at a higher Pa_{O_2}, i.e. oxygen is made available to the tissues more easily.

Oxygen availability is a most important concept to keep in mind during anaesthesia and is summarized by the series of formulae in *Fig.* 2.4.

THE PHARMACOLOGY OF THE INTRAVENOUS ANAESTHETIC AGENTS

Intravenous anaesthetic agents are injected directly into the blood stream where they are carried in the plasma to the tissues. The concentration (or

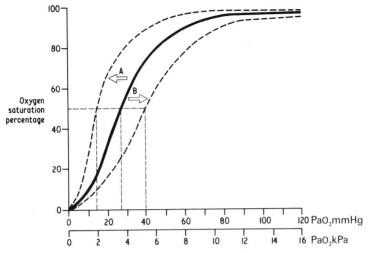

Fig. 2.3. Major influences on the oxygen/haemoglobin dissociation curve. Factors shifting the curve to the left (A) include a fall in body temperature, a fall in the $Paco_2$, increase in blood pH and fall in red cell 2:3 diphosphoglycerate (DPG). The converse of each of these factors is true for shift to the right (B). The horizontal broken line at the 50% O_2 saturation is intersected by the vertical broken lines at the equivalent P_{50}, i.e. the Pao_2 at which the haemoglobin is 50% saturated.

Oxygen availability = Arterial Oxygen Content x Cardiac Output

Arterial Oxygen Content = Oxygen Dissolved in Plasma + Oxygen Carried by Haemoglobin

Oxygen Dissolved in Plasma = 3 ml per litre at 13 kPa & 37°C

Oxygen Carried by Haemoglobin = Haemoglobin Concentration x 1·39* x Percentage Saturation

* *1·39 ml of O_2 are carried by each gram of haemoglobin when fully saturated*

Fig. 2.4. The concept of oxygen availability.

plasma level) of the drug attained during injection causes the agent to diffuse down a concentration gradient across the lipid membranes to the site of action in the brain. The factors which influence the rise and fall of the plasma level of the drug are therefore instrumental in determining the onset of action and recovery from the influence of the agents.

Drugs in Plasma

In the blood all drugs exist either free in the plasma or bound to plasma protein. It is the free drug which provides the effective drug concentration (*see Fig. 2.5*).

The free drug itself can exist in either the ionized or the unionized state and it is only the unionized drug that is lipid soluble and thus able to

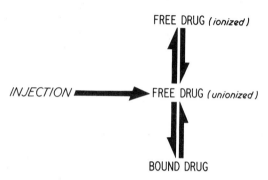

Fig. 2.5. The initial distribution of an intravenously injected drug.

penetrate the lipid membranes to reach the sites of action. Most of the intravenous induction agents are largely unionized. It is theoretically possible for changes in plasma pH to influence the degree of dissociation of the drug into its ions, particularly if the drug is a weak acid, i.e. an alkalosis encouraging ionization of weakly acidic drugs and an acidosis encouraging ionization of weakly alkaline drugs. However, in practice the influence of the drug dose and rate of injection with largely unionized intravenous induction agents renders considerations of pH of minor importance.

As only the unionized unbound drug is lipid soluble it is also this fraction which will be responsible for redistribution into body fat, and uptake and metabolism by the liver (*see Fig. 2.6*).

Onset of Action of the Intravenous Agents

Following intravenous injection the rise in plasma level of the drug is virtually instantaneous and, as all the intravenous anaesthetic agents are highly lipid soluble (i.e. they cross the blood capillary membranes of the blood-brain barrier very easily), the onset of action starts within one arm-to-brain circulation time. The agent travels in the venous drainage from the site of injection in the arm to the right side of the heart and through the pulmonary circulation to the left side of the heart. It is then pumped into the systemic circulation in the arterial blood to reach the brain.

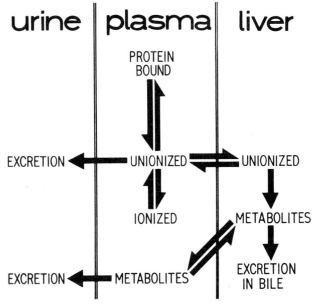

Fig. 2.6. The redistribution, metabolism and excretion of injected drugs. The fat redistribution (although an important factor in drug activity) is not shown.

There are several factors which influence the level to which the plasma concentration rises.

1. The total dose: The greater the dose of drug injected, the higher will be the possible plasma level of drug attained.
2. The duration of the injection: The shorter the injection time, the higher will be the plasma level, as less dilution in the blood will have occurred.
3. The cardiac output: A high cardiac output with a fast circulation time will bring about a more rapid mixing of the drug in the total blood volume and hence the lower will be the plasma level of the drug. This again supports clinical experience, namely that it takes a larger dose of intravenous anaesthetic to put to sleep an agitated, excited patient than would be required to anaesthetize a calm, relaxed patient.
4. The circulating blood volume: The converse of the first factor mentioned above. The smaller the blood volume the greater is the plasma concentration.

Although diffusion of the drug into the extracellular and intracellular compartments rapidly increases the volume into which the drug is distributed, situations in which the blood volume is acutely decreased, e.g. haemorrhagic shock, require careful readjustment of drug dosage in order to avoid overdosage.

Recovery

Recovery from the intravenous anaesthetic agents usually occurs by redistribution of the agent from the central nervous system into the body fat. The initial peak plasma concentration forces the drug into the tissues which are well perfused, i.e. those tissues such as brain, heart, liver and kidneys which have a generous blood supply. Although the adipose tissue is less well perfused by blood, its mass, combined with the high solubility of the anaesthetic agents in fat, causes an increasing amount of the anaesthetic agent to be taken up into the fat stores. This results in a reversal of the blood to brain concentration gradient for the drug, which then moves out of the brain back into the blood allowing the patient to wake up. Assuming that no metabolism takes place, then lipid solubility will be the sole factor influencing recovery. However, metabolism does also influence recovery and provides a further means of reducing the blood level of active drug.

INDIVIDUAL ANAESTHETIC AGENTS

The barbiturates as a group were synthesized in 1903. The basic ring structure is formed by combining urea and malonic acid with the removal of two molecules of water (*see Fig. 2.7*).

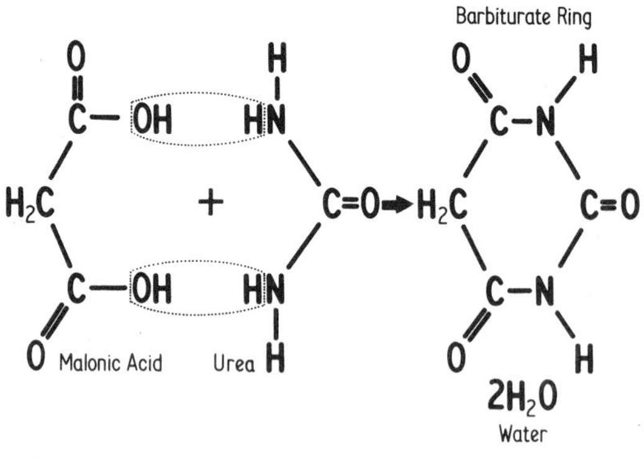

Fig. 2.7. Condensation of one molecule of malonic acid with one molecule of urea to form the barbiturate ring. Two molecules of water are removed in the process.

Modification of the side chain radicals, attached to the carbon atoms, alters the anaesthetic properties presumably by affecting lipid solubility. Currently two drugs are in clinical use as intravenous anaesthetic induction agents.

Thiopentone, introduced in 1934, is the oldest and remains the most widely used intravenous induction agent available. It is a sulphur-containing barbiturate and is available in either single dose 500 mg or multiple dose 2·5 g vials as a yellow powder in an atmosphere of nitrogen. The powder also contains sodium carbonate 6% and when made up in a 2·5% solution it is highly alkaline (pH 10·5), to prevent acid hydrolysis of the barbiturate. In spite of the high pH of the solution, thiopentone is essentially non-irritant on intravenous injection, although it has produced ischaemia on intra-arterial injection, particularly when a 5% solution has been used. Intra-arterial injection has usually resulted following selection of an inappropriate injection site, namely the basilic vein in the medial half of the antecubital fossa overlying the elbow joint and the brachial artery (see Chapter 5).

The drug is highly lipid soluble, a dose of 3–5 mg/kg reliably produces hypnosis in one arm-to-brain circulation time. As a potent central nervous system depressant, transient apnoea will often be seen during induction. It is also a potent cardiovascular depressant and produces a fall in blood pressure, a tachycardia, a fall in the cardiac output and a fall in peripheral vascular resistance. Some care is therefore required in patients with cardiac disease. Adverse reactions, other than the manifestation of relative overdosage, are relatively rare particularly when one considers the millions of anaesthetics induced worldwide per annum with thiopentone.

Sleep time with a single induction dose is of the order of 6–8 min and recovery is by redistribution of the drug from the central nervous system by uptake into body fat. Complete clearance of the drug by liver metabolism and urinary excretion takes up to 48 h and the drug can still be detected in small amounts in the blood 24 h after a single dose. Repeated dosage tends to saturate the fat depot and results in prolonged recovery. For this reason, and the fact that the drug is not stable in aqueous solution (i.e. multidose vials of solution should not be used after 48 h has elapsed), the drug is not popular in dental outpatient anaesthesia.

The second commonly used barbiturate is methohexitone, a non-sulphur-containing sodium methylated oxybarbiturate which was introduced in 1957. It is available in 500 mg multidose vials, containing 30 g sodium carbonate, as a white powder which is dissolved in water in a 1% solution having a pH of 10–11. This solution is stable for several weeks at room temperature. Induction of anaesthesia with methohexitone is rapid, with sleep occurring in one arm-to-brain circulation time using a dose of 1–1·5 mg/kg. Most patients experience some discomfort on injection and some complain of pain at, and proximal to, the site of the injection. The incidence of unwanted side-effects such as hiccough, tremor and muscle movements is higher than with thiopentone, but the cardiovascular depression is said to be less severe. Methohexitone produces a shorter sleep time than thiopentone and the recovery from repeated doses is rather better than with thiopentone. This is probably due to the more rapid metabolism of methohexitone. In spite of the apparently better recovery and lack of hangover following methohexitone anaesthesia, functional impairment of the central nervous system can be demonstrated for up to

24 h. Patients must therefore be firmly discouraged from driving or operating machinery for 24 h following anaesthesia.

Non-barbiturate Anaesthetics

Althesin is a mixture of two steroids, alphaxalone 9 mg/ml and alphadolone 3 mg/ml dissolved with Cremophor EL (a macrogol ester) in 0·25% saline. It is available in single dose 5-ml or 10-ml ampoules and is a rather viscous solution. It is non-irritant on injection with a low incidence of thrombophlebitis and induces sleep in one to two arm-to-brain circulation times with a dose of 0·05–0·1 ml/kg (3–5 ml). Althesin itself causes cardiovascular depression similar to that caused by the barbiturates. However, severe adverse drug reactions are much more common with this agent and include cardiovascular collapse with hypotension and bronchospasm. The sleep time is rather longer than with the barbiturates but repeated doses can be used as metabolism plays a substantial role in the complete recovery from anaesthesia with this drug. The agent possesses no intrinsic steroid activity in the body and is rapidly metabolized by the liver. Althesin possesses advantages as an induction agent for outpatient procedures but the high incidence of severe reactions has limited its use.

Etomidate is a relatively new intravenous anaesthetic induction agent introduced in the mid-1970s. It is available in single dose 10-ml ampoules, dissolved in propylene glycol, having a pH of 8·0. It has a high lipid solubility and is rapidly redistributed into the body fat. The onset of sleep following intravenous injection occurs in one to two arm-to-brain circulation times and the sleep time is 4–5 min with a dose of 0·3 mg/kg. Pain at the site of injection is common. Metabolism by the liver is rapid and 50% of an administered dose is excreted in the urine within 4 h of administration.

The influence of etomidate upon the cardiovascular system appears less marked than with the other intravenous induction agents, with only minor changes in cardiac output and blood pressure being recorded. Spontaneous muscle movements and tremor are common following intravenous injection. Venous thrombosis occurs occasionally.

The advantages of this agent appear to lie in its lack of cardiovascular depression and in its rapid metabolism. However, the drawbacks of pain on injection, spontaneous movement on induction and high cost mitigate against its widespead use.

Propanidid is a eugenol derivative dissolved in Cremophor EL. It is available in 10-ml ampoules containing 500 mg. Its high level of plasma protein binding render rapid injection necessary in order to provide sufficient unbound drug on injection, but thrombophlebitis is uncommon.

The drug has moderate cardiovascular depressant properties (increased by the need for rapid injection) and adverse reactions involving cardiovascular collapse have been frequent enough to virtually relegate the agent from use. It also causes some central nervous system excitation and hyperventilation is a feature of induction with this agent which makes blind nasal intubation a possibility. The drug is quickly metabolized by serum cholinesterase and recovery is rapid and free of hangover, although excitement sometimes occurs.

Ketamine is one of the phencyclidine groups of drugs which can be used to induce anaesthesia. It is a dissociation anaesthetic producing analgesia, amnesia and dissociation from one's surroundings, though the eyes usually remain open. It is painless on injection with a rapid onset of action, causing an increase in cardiac output and blood pressure, with a high incidence of spontaneous movements. The agent has found a use in shocked patients requiring emergency surgery and in the frail, the very young and the very old. However, a very high incidence of nightmares during recovery renders the agent less than ideal for use in dental surgery, most patients finding the visit itself enough of a nightmare!

The fact that the search for an 'ideal' intravenous induction agent continues, indicates that all the available agents have some drawbacks. Recent interest has focused on the newer benzodiazepines, in particular on midazolam, which is water soluble and has a plasma half-life of about 2 h (i.e. about one-tenth that of diazepam). In spite of the promise of such agents, namely much reduced cardiovascular depression combined with potent sedation, the long half-life and the high dosage required to induce anaesthesia result in prolonged postoperative drowsiness which is unacceptable in outpatient practice. It is curious to note that the two barbiturate agents introduced between 30 and 50 years ago still hold clinical preference.

The clinical application of these agents is discussed in Chapter 5 and the pharmacology of the hypnosedatives is outlined in Chapter 6. It is important that the principles described in this chapter are understood for it is in their application that sound clinical practice and judgement must be based.

CHAPTER 3

INHALATION ANAESTHESIA

Inhalation anaesthesia remains the commonest form of general anaesthesia for dental extractions in the UK with more than one million anaesthetics of this type administered each year. Before 1956 there were various methods of inducing anaesthesia by inhalation. Rapid induction of anaesthesia could be achieved but with a definite risk of an increased morbidity and mortality. For example, one could use 100% nitrous oxide with consequent hypoxia or a potent volatile agent such as chloroform or ethyl chloride with the risk of fatal cardiac arrhythmias. Alternatively, one could choose the rather slower induction offered by ether, avoiding hypoxia but often entailing a stormy induction and recovery with the added unpleasant side effect of vomiting.

The introduction of halothane in 1956 and its subsequent widespread clinical use has rendered the use of hypoxic anaesthetic mixtures totally unnecessary, and has removed almost completely the risk of a fatal arrhythmia occurring during induction. Similarly the incidence of postoperative vomiting has been greatly reduced with the modern inhalational agents.

Induction of anaesthesia will be considered in the context of the modern inhalational agents and their effects on the respiratory and cardiovascular systems. Maintenance of anaesthesia and postoperative recovery are also discussed and the final section deals with anaesthetic equipment.

INDUCTION OF INHALATION ANAESTHESIA

Inhalation anaesthesia is still preferred by many practitioners who feel uneasy about the rapid loss of consciousness and depressed airway reflexes obtained with the intravenous agents. It is often, if rather surprisingly, preferred by patients brought up in terror of the needle.

Classically, inhalation anaesthesia has been described as occurring in four stages, the definition of the stages being based on the changes in the eyes, the respiration and reflexes which are induced in the patient by the anaesthetic agent and observed as the signs of anaesthesia. Guedel was the first to define clearly the stages in terms of the signs and his work was based on ether anaesthesia. Although induction with the modern inhalation agents is much more rapid than with ether, and therefore the stages of anaesthesia are passed through much more rapidly, sufficient signs of the classic inhalation anaesthesia are seen with modern inhalation agents to warrant description of the stages.

INHALATION ANAESTHESIA

Stage I

The stage of analgesia in which the patient becomes analgesic and disorientated. It persists until loss of consciousness when it is no longer possible to communicate with the patient. In this stage the respiration is rapid and may be irregular, the pupils are small with eye co-ordination gradually lost as the second stage supervenes and consciousness is lost.

Stage II

The excitement stage persists from the loss of consciousness until rhythmical respiration is restored. In the days of ether anaesthesia this stage was often associated with violent struggling and shouting by the patient. Communication with the patient is lost, the breathing pattern is rapid and irregular, the pupils are large and the eyes may diverge and show spontaneous movement. The eyelash reflex is still present.

Stage III

The stage of surgical anaesthesia is associated with the onset of regular respiration and loss of eyelash reflex. The pupils remain small, but some spontaneous eye movements still occur. Surgical anaesthesia is described as having four planes with increasing depth of anaesthesia from plane I to plane IV. There is an associated increase of voluntary muscle flaccidity, respiratory depression, pupillary dilatation with fixed central gaze and the loss of the laryngeal reflexes. Resort to the deeper planes of surgical anaesthesia as evidenced by respiratory depression, fixed central gaze and pupillary dilatation is rarely, if ever, required in oral surgery.

Stage IV

The patient becomes apnoeic due to medullary paralysis. This constitutes an anaesthetic accident and should never be allowed to occur.

Occasionally apnoea occurs during the excitement phase of Stage II but this can be easily differentiated from medullary paralysis as the eyelash reflex will still be present and the eyes will be divergent and moving.

Stage I anaesthesia is discussed more fully in Chapter 4 and the features of the later stages are outlined in *Fig.* 3.1.

Induction of anaesthesia must always have been preceded by an interview with the patient in which the anaesthetic history is reviewed. This interview should be carried out by the anaesthetist himself or by a colleague with an appropriate knowledge of the factors influencing a general anaesthetic. It is the duty of all practitioners to establish who is responsible for this interview.

The patient should then be positioned comfortably in the dental chair in such a way as to facilitate both the contemplated surgery and the

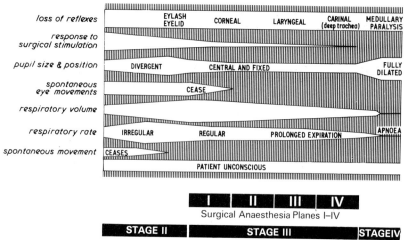

Fig. 3.1. Diagram to illustrate Guedel's stages of anaesthesia, modified for use with the modern inhalational agents (cf. *Fig.* 4.1).

administration of the anaesthetic. There are two basic positions in which the procedure can be carried out, either sitting up or lying down.

There is some controversy over which position is associated with the lower morbidity.

The Sitting-up Position

This is the traditional dental chair posture, which still retains advantages for both surgery and anaesthesia.

1. In the erect posture the floor of the mouth slopes downwards from the posterior part to the anterior part of the oral cavity. This is clearly demonstrated in *Fig.* 3.12. This encourages debris such as saliva, blood, pus or amalgam etc. to gravitate to the anterior part of the oral cavity from whence it can be aspirated, thus decreasing the risk of debris contaminating the oropharynx and larynx with the possibility of laryngospasm or aspiration into the lungs.

2. The patient's head is at a more advantageous working level for the operator, and the anaesthetist can assist the operator for instance in extraction of upper teeth when the firm upward pressure on the maxilla exerted by the forceps can be counteracted by the anaesthetist controlling head movement by downward pressure on the vertex of the skull.

3. With the patient sitting up maintenance of a patent airway is marginally easier for the anaesthetist as gravity assists in keeping the mandible forwards and slightly downwards.

4. Spontaneous respiration requires less effort in the sitting-up position. When erect, gravity pulls the abdominal contents downwards away from

the diaphragm making the upward and downward excursion of diaphragmatic movement easier. This improvement in respiratory compliance reduces the work of breathing.

5. Gravity will also encourage the gastric contents (hopefully very little) to remain at the lower end of the oesophagus, where they belong, thus reducing the risk of silent regurgitation of gastric acid into the oropharynx with subsequent aspiration into the lungs. Prior to the widespread adoption of Sellick's manoeuvre (cricoid cartilage pressure) during induction of emergency anaesthesia, the sitting-up position was adopted during induction of emergency cases suspected of having a full stomach.

The points against the sitting position during anaesthesia and surgery are as follows:

1. The return of venous blood to the heart from the lower half of the body will be hindered by gravity and pooling of blood in the veins of the lower limbs will occur. This reduction in venous return will cause a fall in cardiac output leading to a fall in the blood pressure.

2. The vertical distance between the level of the brain and the level of the heart will cause a pressure gradient to exist between the two. Thus the blood pressure produced at the heart level will be reduced at the head level. Both points (1) and (2) have been cited as the cause of fainting during anaesthesia with the possibility of consequent ischaemic brain damage.

Elevating the legs and feet will help to improve venous return with a reduced risk of a major fall in blood pressure (*Fig.* 3.2). Maintenance of an adequate perfusion pressure in the erect posture will also be helped by avoidance of high concentrations of the potent inhalational agents, and by careful patient selection, avoiding extremes of age and those with disorders of cardiac function.

3. Should debris from the oral cavity be allowed to slip backwards over the base of the tongue into the oropharynx, gravity will encourage it to fall directly into the larynx with resultant coughing, laryngospasm and possible soiling of the lungs. The likelihood of this occurring will be reduced if the floor of the mouth is maintained sloping downwards from back to front. Over extension of the neck during induction will raise the mentum of the mandible causing debris to run backwards along the floor of the mouth towards the base of the tongue.

The Recumbent Supine or Lying Position

This is now used increasingly for procedures under general anaesthesia, particularly if the patient is intubated. Its advantages are:

1. Venous return from the lower limbs is unimpeded, and cardiac output and blood pressure are therefore better maintained.

2. A perfusion pressure gradient does not exist between the head and the heart.

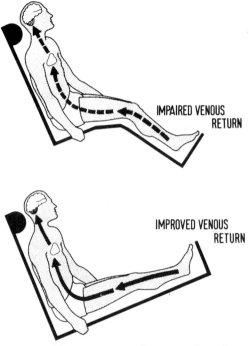

Fig. 3.2. Improvement in venous return and consequently cardiac output with elevation of the legs.

3. The operator and the anaesthetist can sit down to carry out many procedures. (This may have the disadvantage of removing any sense of urgency to complete the procedure.)

The disadvantages are:

1. The abdominal contents can now press against the diaphragm with the possibility of producing respiratory embarrassment. Spontaneous respiration costs more work in the supine position.

2. Fluid and solid debris can fall directly backwards into the oropharynx. However, proponents of the supine position would argue that the foreign matter can be seen easily and immediately aspirated and furthermore gravity does not encourage debris to fall into the larynx and lungs in this position.

Having suitably positioned the patient and checked the equipment, induction of anaesthesia can now begin. The anaesthetist must *always* check his machine and ancillary equipment both before and during use.

Most patients are rather nervous during the induction of anaesthesia and it helps to be able to establish a rapport with the patient before the inhalation commences. Only the anaesthetist should talk to the patient during induction, especially if the patient is apprehensive, or a child. Two or three people talking at once in an attempt to reassure the patient only increases his or her apprehension.

Assuming that a nose mask is to be used it must be explained to the patient that he or she must breathe normally through the nose. It helps to have checked the patency of the nasal airway by asking the patient to take a few deep breaths through the nose, prior to commencing the induction.

The inspired mixture of gases from the anaesthetic machine should consist of a minimum of 30% oxygen (O_2) in nitrous oxide (N_2O) 70%. Many modern machines will now automatically deliver this minimum oxygen concentration as a built-in safety mechanism prevents the delivery of mixtures containing less. The flow rate of the mixture required will need to be adjusted according to which circuit is in use.

The nasal or face mask should be gently applied to the patient's nose or face while the anaesthetist quietly explains the procedure to the patient (*Fig.* 3.3). As the uptake and onset of action of nitrous oxide is rapid, the potent inhalation agent, either halothane or enflurane, can be introduced into the inspired mixture in low concentration immediately in most patients. However, the euphoric effects of eight to ten breaths of the N_2O/O_2 mixture prior to the introduction of the potent agent will render

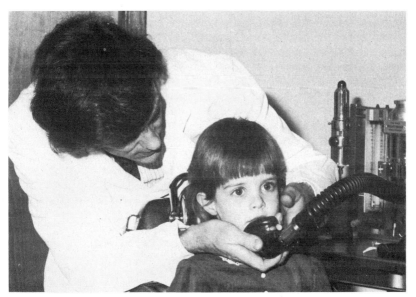

Fig. 3.3. Gentle application of the mask to the face. The position of the anaesthetist's hands effectively extends the mask and allows control of the patient's head in case of restlessness. The anaesthetist must attempt to distract the patient by quietly maintaining a continuous patter of conversation. (A talking patient *has* to breathe!)

the obnoxious smell more acceptable to the nervous patient. Communication with the patient should be maintained for as long as possible, the anaesthetist quietly reassuring the patient as the induction proceeds. Silence and decorum should be maintained by the operative team during induction as this renders a smooth induction more likely (*Fig.* 3.4).

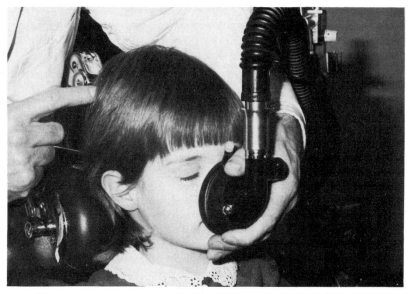

Fig. 3.4. The patient asleep. Control of the patient's head can be achieved with a hand as shown using the little finger to support the chin.

The effective monitoring of clinical signs during the induction of anaesthesia need not involve sophisticated equipment. However, total attention to the patient is required as induction of anaesthesia will profoundly influence the respiratory and cardiovascular systems. It is a clear airway, however, which is the cornerstone of safe inhalation anaesthesia. Anatomically (using a nasal mask) the airway extends from the nares via the nasal cavity, through the nasopharynx, oropharynx, larynx, trachea, bronchi and bronchioles (*Fig.* 3.5). Obstruction can occur at any of these sites and is potentially the most dangerous mishap to occur in anaesthesia.

Nasal obstruction occurs with upper respiratory tract infection, deviated nasal septa (usually post-traumatic), hay fever (common in spring and early summer) and nasal polypi (common in people working in dusty environments). The nasal airway must always be formally assessed pre-induction. Nasal obstruction can usually be relieved during induction by

INHALATION ANAESTHESIA

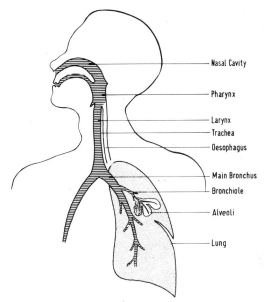

Fig. 3.5. Diagrammatic representation of the various sections of the airway.

the insertion of a Silastic rubber nasal airway, well lubricated with a sterile water soluble jelly. This manoeuvre markedly improves nasal breathing and only rarely is a cause of epistaxis. Such an airway cannot be inserted while the patient is awake.

The nasopharynx is occasionally a site of airway obstruction in children with enlarged tonsils and adenoids, and concurrent infection will aggravate this situation.

Obstruction of the airway in the oropharynx is the commonest problem seen in clinical practice. During induction loss of muscle tone in the soft tissues of the floor of the mouth allows the tongue to slip backwards into the oropharynx, causing it to impinge on the soft palate and posterior oropharyngeal wall. Over flexion of the neck causes upward pressure to be exerted on the base of the tongue forcing it into the airway, thereby causing obstruction.

Thus, during induction, the most common causes of airway obstruction can be relieved by appropriate attention to the mandible and neck. Moderate flexion of the neck combined with forward pressure on the mandible enables the oropharyngeal airway optimal dimensions in the sagittal plane by keeping the soft tissues of the floor of the mouth out of the airway (*Fig.* 3.6). Pressure on the mandible must be applied from behind the ramus avoiding any pressure from beneath the mandible which would cause upward and backward movement of the tongue into the

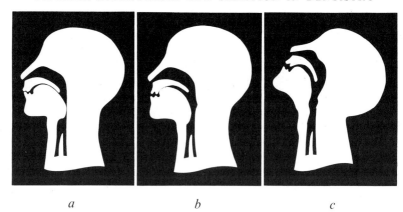

Fig. 3.6. Diagrammatic representation of the airway dimensions (cf. page 45). In *a* the airway is virtually obstructed. In *b* it has been improved by forward protrusion of the mandible while in *c* a further improvement is obtained by extending the head on the atlanto-occipital joint.

oropharynx. This is particularly important in children in whom the physical dimensions of the airway are reduced.

Laryngeal obstruction during induction of anaesthesia can be due to laryngospasm or solid foreign bodies becoming lodged at the level of the vocal cords. Laryngospasm is not uncommon in the sitting-up position particularly if the neck has been hyperextended in an attempt to improve or maintain the airway. With hyperextension of the neck the floor of the mouth no longer runs forwards and downwards and any liquid matter in the mouth, usually saliva, then runs backwards over the base of the tongue falling directly down towards the laryngeal inlet, initiating the laryngospasm by which means the reflexes attempt to protect the lungs from soiling by foreign matter. The incidence of laryngospasm is reduced in calm patients due to lower levels of salivary secretions. The timely use of oral suction during induction and avoiding hyperextension of the neck may also reduce its incidence.

Mechanical obstruction of the larynx by solid matter is more unusual, but has been caused by prostheses. Obstruction of the major airways below the cords, i.e. the larynx and main bronchi, can occur should a large foreign body, e.g. a porcelain crown, manage to slip past the vocal cords. More commonly obstruction below the cords occurs in the small airways due to either secretions as in bronchitis or bronchospasm as in asthma. A mixed picture of obstruction due to solid particles, secretions and bronchospasm may be seen in cases of aspiration of gastric content (Mendelson's Syndrome).

INHALATION ANAESTHESIA

Signs of Airway Obstruction

Airway obstruction influences the observable signs of respiration by:
1. Altering the mechanics of breathing.
2. Adversely affecting the gas exchange in the lungs.
3. Affecting gas flow in the anaesthetic circuit.

Alterations in the breathing mechanisms depend upon whether the site of obstruction is situated above or below the vocal cords, and the features of each need separate consideration.

Alterations in the Mechanics of Breathing

The variations which occur as consequences of airway obstruction are directly dependent on the site of obstruction. This may be either at or above the vocal cords or below the vocal cords.

During quiet breathing the intermittent contraction in concert of the diaphragm and the intercostal muscles and their subsequent relaxation produces a gentle rise and fall of the chest wall and abdomen. The movement of the anterior chest and abdominal wall is in phase, i.e. they move up and down together. During obstruction of the upper airway, the air or anaesthetic gases are prevented from entering the lungs during inspiration. In spite of the lack of airflow into the lungs, the diaphragm and intercostal muscles continue to attempt to increase the volume of the thorax; the diaphragm by pulling downwards increasing the superior–inferior dimensions, and the intercostal muscles by pulling upwards and outwards, increasing the width and the anterior–posterior dimensions of the chest. These forces exerted by the respiratory muscles during inspiration against the obstructed airway will cause a large fall in the intrathoracic pressure which cannot be translated into the normal volume change of an inspired breath. As the diaphragm is the stronger of the muscle groups involved, it will overcome the action of the intercostal muscles and as the diaphragm moves downwards will cause the chest wall to move downwards and inwards on inspiration. Because this movement of the chest wall is the reverse of that anticipated during inspiration it is called paradoxical respiration. The descriptive term 'see-saw respiration' is also applied to describe the relative movements of the chest wall and abdominal wall during airway obstruction as on inspiration the chest moves in and the abdomen moves out and vice versa on expiration (*Fig.* 3.7).

The imbalance in chest wall movement will be detected by stretch receptors in the intercostal muscles and relayed to the respiratory centre via the spinal cord. This will result in an increasing respiratory drive being applied to the muscles of respiration and the accessory muscles of respiration, e.g. the strap muscles of the neck will be recruited in an effort to maintain tidal exchange. The combined effect of this respiratory muscle activity during the induction of anaesthesia can produce the impression that the patient is fighting for breath, which indeed he is!

Partial airway obstruction will allow some airflow into the chest but the signs of altered chest wall mechanics will be similar to, although less marked than, total airway obstruction. It is usual for airflow past an obstruction to make a noise, and in partial airway obstruction the sounds of partial strangulation accompany the normal breathing pattern. Less severe obstruction may be accompanied merely by snoring noises. Airway obstruction above the cords almost always influences the mechanics of inspiration.

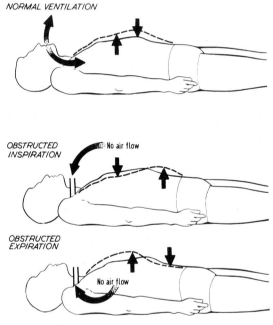

Fig. 3.7. Paradoxical (see-saw) respiration.

Obstruction below the vocal cords differs from upper airway obstruction in two important aspects. Firstly, the obstruction tends to be diffuse, i.e. not concentrated at one point, but distributed among the small airways, e.g. retention of secretions, bronchitis and bronchospasm. Secondly, the obstruction lies within the thoracic cavity and is therefore influenced by the changes in intrathoracic pressure during the respiratory cycle. This second effect means that during inspiration the fall in intrathoracic pressure is pulling outward on the small airways, i.e. tending to enlarge them and during expiration the rise in intrathoracic pressure is acting to compress the small airways and reduce their diameter. This increases the airways resistance during expiration, i.e. it is harder to breathe out, and a prolonged expiratory phase is seen. Once again proprioceptors in the chest wall detect the decrease in compliance during expiration, the information is relayed to the respiratory centre in the brain stem, and drive is applied to the muscles of respiration to assist expiration. Thus, expiration which is normally passive, i.e. the chest wall and lungs normally fall back to their resting position on expiration, becomes active as the patient attempts to force the expired air past the small airway obstruction. As the expired gases whistle through the small airways an expiratory wheeze is produced.

Adverse Effects on Gas Exchange

Airway obstruction adversely influences gas exchange in the lungs which will produce changes in the observed clinical signs during induction.

Impaired oxygen delivery to the alveoli during obstruction will result in a lowered partial pressure of oxygen in the blood resulting in cyanosis. A healthy patient becomes rapidly cyanosed during complete airway obstruction but cyanosis may take several minutes to develop in less severe cases of upper and lower airway obstruction. Associated with such periods of hypoxia will be a marked increase in the patient's heart rate and a sharp rise in blood pressure.

Carbon dioxide clearance from the blood will be impeded during obstruction with a resultant increase in the partial pressure of carbon dioxide in the blood. This, in turn, provides a strong stimulus to the respiratory centre which responds by increasing the respiratory rate and the depth of respiration. As the obstruction will effectively prevent any increase in the depth of respiration, strenuous activity of the respiratory muscles will be noted as the outcome of this situation. The increase in respiratory rate must be differentiated from the transient increase in respiratory rate seen during the brief excitement phase of a normal inhalation induction.

The rise in Pa_{CO_2} will also augment the rise in heart rate and blood pressure seen with hypoxia. In addition, the increase in endogenous catecholamine secretion produced by the hypoxia and hypercapnoea will, if halothane is being used, lead to cardiac arrhythmias with a rapid and irregular heart beat. Perspiration in the absence of surgical stimulation should also be regarded as a sign of carbon dioxide retention.

Uptake of the anaesthetic agent will be impaired by the inefficient gas exchange during airway obstruction. This will increase the time taken to induce the patient and may cause an increase in the length of the excitation stage. Airway obstruction must therefore be suspected when a patient exhibits an unusually long period of excitement during induction.

GENERAL ANAESTHESIA AND SEDATION IN DENTISTRY

Alterations of Gas Flow in the Anaesthetic Circuit

The two circuits in common use are the Magill, with its modifications, and the Bain circuit (*see* p. 66). During normal, unobstructed respiration via the circuits observation of the reservoir bag and listening to the sounds made by the expiratory valve will provide further indication of normal or obstructed respiration.

Unobstructed inspiration produces a peak inspiratory flow rate of about 30 litres/min, and, as the fresh gas flow rate depending upon the circuit used will be of the order of 5–10 litres/min, the deficit is taken from the reservoir bag. If there is a good mask fit around the nose or face the reservoir bag will be seen to partially deflate during inspiration. This partial deflation is inadequate or totally absent if the patient's respiration is shallow or obstructed. Sudden release of the mask fit on the face will also produce a similar partial deflation of the bag. In total airway obstruction the subatmospheric pressure in the chest during inspiration fails to reach the anaesthetic circuit and the bag remains inflated. Careful attention to the noises produced by the expiratory valve will provide additional information during obstruction as the fresh gas flow, having filled the reservoir bag, will spill past the expiratory valve keeping the valve continuously open.

Management of Airway Obstruction

Early detection and correction of airway obstruction is essential to prevent the development of the sequence hypoxia—cardiac arrhythmias—cardiac arrest. Undetected airway obstruction is the prime cause of most dental anaesthetic accidents. The specific measures to relieve the obstruction will be dictated by the site at which it occurs.

Nasal obstruction can usually be relieved during induction by the insertion of a Silastic rubber nasal airway, well lubricated with a sterile water soluble jelly. This manoeuvre markedly improves nasal breathing and only rarely is it the cause of epistaxis. Such an airway, however, cannot be inserted when the patient is awake.

Oropharyngeal obstruction, the commonest site, can be relieved by appropriate attention to the mandible and the neck. Modest flexion of the neck combined with some extension of the head on the atlanto-occipital joint will relieve any downward pressure on the floor of the mouth and displacement of the mandible anteriorly on the temporo-mandibular joint will move the soft tissues attached to the mandible forwards out of the oropharynx, thus providing optimal airway dimensions in the sagittal plane. The pressure on the mandible (*Fig.* 3.8) must be applied from behind the ramus avoiding any pressure from beneath the mandible into the floor of the mouth which would cause upward and backward movement of the tongue into the oropharynx. This is particularly important in children in whom the physical dimensions of the airway are reduced.

INHALATION ANAESTHESIA

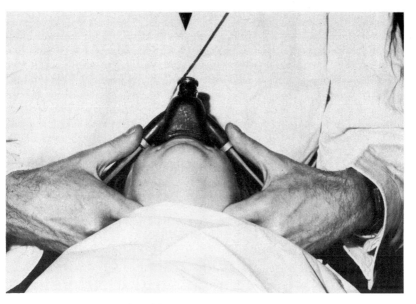

Fig. 3.8. The application of forward pressure on the mandible by positioning the knuckle of the index finger behind the ramus.

Laryngospasm is a common complication during an inhalation dental anaesthetic, the varying severity of which will indicate the appropriate management. Mild laryngospasm, in which the patient phonates or makes crowing noises, but maintains respiratory exchange, can be treated merely by performing oropharyngeal toilet, aspirating any liquid matter to prevent further stimulation of the laryngeal reflexes by contamination from the oral cavity. This, in conjunction with attention to the general airway anatomy, will usually resolve the problem.

Moderately severe laryngospasm, in which the patient's respiratory exchange is reduced, will require the above measures, but an increase in the inspired oxygen concentration will also be required in order to maintain oxygen uptake. In addition, it may be necessary to remove all instrumentation from the patient's mouth, to clear the upper airway completely and allow the laryngospasm to resolve before continuing with the surgery. Positive airway pressure applied manually from the reservoir bag will also aid air entry during inspiration.

Severe laryngospasm, in which there is no entry of air into the lungs, must be treated as an emergency. Oxygenation must be attempted by the use of 100% oxygen and positive pressure artificial respiration must be applied using the reservoir bag in synchronization with the patient's own respiratory efforts. A full face mask will be more effective in giving an airtight seal in order to be able to effectively achieve artificial ventilation. If a foreign body at the vocal cords is suspected as the cause of the obstruction or laryngospasm, then laryngoscopy and clearing the airway with Magill's forceps or suction will be required. Should it prove impossible to oxygenate the patient, cricothyrotomy with a large bore needle will give a ready route for oxygen administration using plastic tubing and a Y connector (*Fig.* 3.9). However, laryngoscopy and intubation would be a more conventional approach with the use of a depolarizing muscle relaxant to overcome the laryngospasm, but every attempt must be made to oxygenate the patient prior to attempting intubation. This is not a technique to attempt without adequate experience in controlled intubation.

Acute airway obstruction below the cords, in the lower respiratory tract, is most commonly situated in the small airways, e.g. acute asthmatic bronchospasm. General measures aimed at maintaining oxygenation must

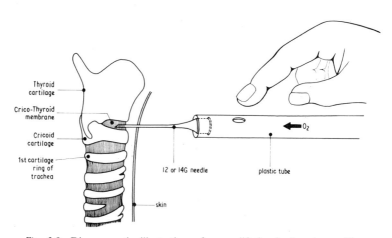

Fig. 3.9. Diagrammatic illustration of a modified cricothyrotomy. The importance of the hole in the plastic tubing cannot be understated as it forms a T-piece anaesthetic circuit and allows positive pressure ventilation by intermittently occluding the hole. It also prevents over inflation of the lungs.

be combined with specific therapy to decrease the bronchomotor tone and relieve the spasm. Both halothane and enflurane are efficient bronchodilators and bronchospasm, which is unusual during dental anaesthesia, usually responds favourably to the potent inhalational agents. Specific bronchodilators such as aminophylline, salbutamol and adrenaline can be administered by injection, but great caution is required when giving these agents as they interact with halothane on the myocardium to produce arrhythmias.

A foreign body causing airway obstruction below the cords is a life-threatening emergency and the patient must be transported to hospital while being given 100% oxygen, as bronchoscopy will be required to remove it.

MAINTENANCE

The assessment of the depth of anaesthesia must be made at the same time as the patient's respiration and circulation are being monitored, and a working knowledge of the stages of anaesthesia (*see* p. 39) is essential for this assessment.

As induction proceeds the concentration of inhalational agent administered can be gradually increased from, for example, 0·5% halothane, via 1% to 1·5%. Concentrations of halothane greater than 1·5% inhaled in a 70/30% mixture of nitrous oxide/oxygen are rarely required for straightforward extraction of teeth. Higher concentrations are not accepted as readily by the patient and lead to greater circulatory and respiratory depression with a more prolonged recovery period. Similar considerations apply to enflurane with the added cautionary note that an inspired concentration of twice the MAC of enflurane (*c.* 3·5%) leads to marked depression of the cardiac output resulting in a greater fall in blood pressure than halothane.

The transition point between induction and the maintenance of inhalation anaesthetic is judged to be passed when the following three criteria are met:

1. Regular respiration is established.
2. There is no eyelash reflex.
3. The mouth can be opened without undue force to allow the insertion of a dental prop.

Both regular respiration and absence of the eyelash reflex are signs of the establishment of stage III, plane I surgical anaesthesia while it is necessary as a purely practical point to be able to open the mouth to carry out the procedure. Spontaneous eye movement is seen at this depth of anaesthesia and this must not be confused with the presence or absence of the eyelash reflex.

During the maintenance of the anaesthetic the anaesthetist must not only monitor all the vital functions which were observed during induction, but must also co-operate with the operator to achieve optimum surgical access while at the same time ensuring that the manoeuvres employed in achieving access and packing of the oral cavity do not cause airway obstruction.

The prop, the pack or the operator's fingers can all lead to airway obstruction during the procedure. Insertion of the prop, in order to open the mouth, will cause the soft tissues of the base of the tongue to move backwards and downwards into the airway. A concerted effort by the anaesthetist to ensure adequate forward displacement of the mandible will pull these soft tissues out of the airway.

In all dental procedures it is essential to pack the mouth to provide as much protection as possible to the pharyngeal and laryngeal airways. The mouth pack can, if over vigorously or carelessly inserted, force the soft palate upwards and backwards into the nasopharynx, thus obstructing the airway. Although efficient packing reduces the likelihood of loss of teeth etc. into the pharynx or larynx, care must be taken by the operator not to obstruct the airway in this manner, as there is nothing that the anaesthetist can do to relieve it. These comments apply particularly to children in whom the volume of the oral cavity is small. Gauze packs should be inserted with a view to occluding access to the pharynx from the mouth and to lift the tongue forwards and upwards (*Fig.* 3.10). Correctly used V packs (*Fig.* 3.11) have much to commend them as they not only occlude the mouth but improve the nasopharyngeal dimensions (*Fig.* 3.12).

When at all possible the operator, particularly if extracting lower teeth, must try to exert forward traction on the mandible with his free hand to assist this effort. To achieve this the operator must hold the jaw in a

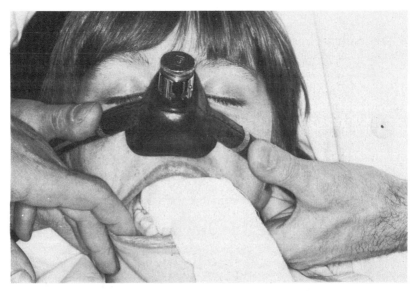

Fig. 3.10. A gauze pack. Correctly placed it should occlude the lingual sulcus and oropharynx while supporting the tongue in a forward position. This should allow an excellent naso-pharyngeal airway. The anaesthetist's hands should be rotated back away from the operative field. Although placed by the surgeon the pack remains the responsibility of the anaesthetist.

INHALATION ANAESTHESIA

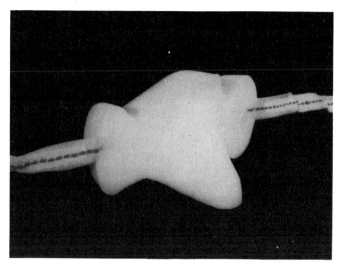

Fig. 3.11. The V pack. It is anatomically designed to provide optimal airway dimensions while completely occluding the oropharynx (cf. *Fig.* 3.12).

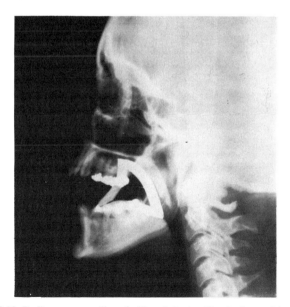

Fig. 3.12. Radio-opaque outline of a V pack *in situ*. The shadows of the nasal, pharyngeal and tracheal airways can be clearly seen.

forward position rather than concentrating on support of the socket which is a secondary consideration during extractions under general anaesthesia. Fingers should not be placed in the lingual sulcus unless it is absolutely necessary, since there is a high risk of airway obstruction caused by the downward displacement of the soft tissues of the floor of the mouth into the oropharynx. Additionally the operator should place a finger under the lower border of the mandible and apply an equal and opposite force to the apical pressure exerted during extraction (*Fig.* 3.13). Extraction of the upper teeth, particularly molars, will render the operator powerless to assist in this way. The mouth needs to be opened as widely as possible to achieve adequate access so special attention must be paid by the anaesthetist when these teeth are being extracted.

Although, in general, these factors involve the operator rather than the anaesthetist, both must pay them close attention to give the best airway management. It is also the responsibility of the team to ensure that adequate oral suction to remove saliva, blood and solid material is carried out during the procedure. This leaves a clean operative field, reducing the risk of both laryngospasm and coughing during the operation and postoperative aspiration of such material into the lungs.

The anaesthetist must also note that when elevators are being used in lower jaw extraction the operator may be unable to adequately support

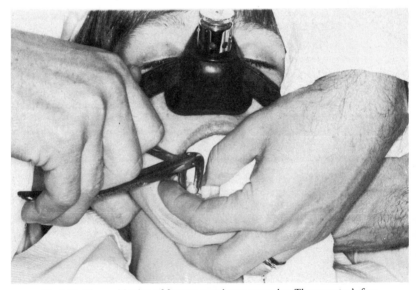

Fig. 3.13. The positioning of forceps on a lower premolar. The operator's free hand should support the mandible in a forward position and apply equal and opposite pressure to the apical pressures exerted during extraction. The thumb should not be pushed back into the lingual sulcus.

INHALATION ANAESTHESIA

the jaw and the risk of displacing the tongue downwards into the airway is greater. This situation requires firm pressure on the ramus of the mandible by the anaesthetist to maintain the airway.

Placement of the anaesthetist's hand during maintenance is also important in securing good surgical access as the operator requires a clear field in front of the face. This entails the anaesthetist maintaining adequate pressure on the tubes supplying the nasal mask to achieve a good mask fit while at the same time rotating the hands backwards and applying appropriate pressure with the knuckles of the index fingers to the ramus (*Fig.* 3.14). This grip on the patient's head maintains control of the airway, permits control of the head and allows the operator uninhibited access to the oral cavity. Control of the head movement will also be needed, for instance in the extraction of upper teeth during which the operator applies upward pressure with the forceps on the maxilla.

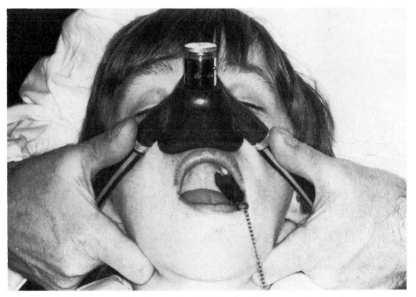

Fig. 3.14. Support of the jaw and mask following placement of a dental prop. The practical details of mouth-opening are not discussed as considerable variations in technique are encountered. Adequate and stable opening of the mouth is an obvious requirement before proceeding operatively.

RECOVERY

A prior knowledge of the number of extractions, their site and possible difficulty will influence the decision, to be made during anaesthesia, when to reduce the inhaled concentration of vapour to initiate recovery.

Recovery is the most dangerous period in dental anaesthesia. The analogy with aircraft travel is often quoted, namely that take off and landing are the dangerous times in a flight. Without a doubt both in air travel and in anaesthesia the return to earth, i.e. recovery, can be very dangerous as the majority of reported accidents occur during this critical phase.

The problems arise because:

1. The potential for airway obstruction is, if anything increased, as foreign matter, i.e. blood, amalgam, etc., is invariably present in the upper airway.

2. The anaesthetist may be pre-occupied with starting the next anaesthetic.

3. The recovery facilities in many locations in which dental anaesthesia takes place are often unsatisfactory.

The risk of a life-threatening episode of airway obstruction during recovery can be reduced by ensuring adequate clearance of debris from the oral cavity, and most importantly by ensuring that the patient is in a fit state to maintain his or her own airway. Adequate supervision is essential until this point is reached. A simple consideration of the facts of uptake and elimination of inhaled general anaesthetics lead to the conclusion that the longer the operative procedure, and the deeper the anaesthesia, the longer will be the recovery phase during which the patient will remain incapable of maintaining a clear airway. Clinical experience and training will develop the judgement required to be able to turn off the anaesthetic vapours at a suitable time prior to the end of the surgical procedure so that recovery is under way when surgery is complete.

An anaesthetic must never be started in a second patient while a previous patient is inadequately recovered, as this compromises the care of both patients. Should a previous patient develop an airway problem while the second patient is being anaesthetized, there will be two patients at risk with only one anaesthetist to manage them. Financial or scheduling pressures must never be allowed to prejudice patient care by causing hurried work.

The minimum recovery facilities available should consist of a tipping trolley or couch upon which the patient can be recovered, an emergency supply of oxygen with a suitable delivery tube and face mask, a suction apparatus with a rigid oropharyngeal suction end and a trained assistant capable of recognizing airway obstruction and dealing with simple airway or circulatory problems.

The patient should be recovered lying on his or her side. This encourages drainage of debris from the mouth, with the face turned downwards (*Fig.* 3.15). This still allows the recovery nurse to observe the patient's colour and respiration and makes maintenance of the airway easier as the soft tissues tend to fall forward towards the front of the mouth. If necessary, the trolley can be tipped into a head-down position

INHALATION ANAESTHESIA

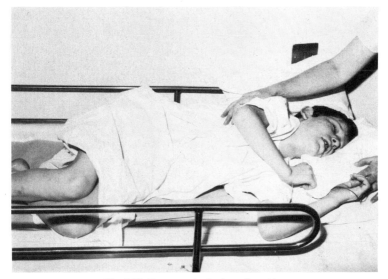

Fig. 3.15. Recovery in the lateral position.

should the patient vomit or bleed profusely into the airway. Prior to allowing the assistant to take over the patient's care, the anaesthetist should ensure that all packs and swabs have been removed from the mouth and that the patient responds purposefully to stimuli. Firm pressure on the cartilage of the ear, just sufficient to elicit a response, should be applied and a suitable response would consist of both a grimace and movement of the patient's hand and arm in an attempt to remove the stimulus. This level of response indicates that the patient has sufficient muscle tone and co-ordination to allow delegation of recovery duty to one's assistant. Further recovery should consist of gradually allowing the patient to sit up and then walk with support. The patient should be able to walk unsupported prior to leaving the recovery area. All patients should be seen by the anaesthetist prior to their leaving, to ascertain their suitability to leave, to ensure that their escort is present and to warn them once more not to drink alcohol, drive a car or operate any machinery for 24 h post-anaesthetic.

EQUIPMENT

The equipment required for administering an inhalation anaesthetic consists of:
  1. A supply of the gases, oxygen and nitrous oxide.

GENERAL ANAESTHESIA AND SEDATION IN DENTISTRY

2. A machine to control the flows of the gases and the concentration of the administered vapour (i.e. a vaporizer designed specifically for halothane or enflurane).

3. A suitable circuit to administer the inhaled mixture to the patient.

Emergency equipment should also be immediately available for intubation and ventilation (Chapter 7).

Supply of Gases

Anaesthetic gases in the UK are supplied in colour coded steel cylinders in standard sizes. The cylinders are inspected and pressure tested at regular intervals by the manufacturer. Those supplied for connection directly to anaesthetic machines are pin indexed. The valve face of the cylinder has two holes drilled into it and the distance between these holes is specific for the type of gas the cylinder contains. Each yoke of the anaesthetic machine to which a cylinder is connected possesses a pair of pins designed to fit into the holes in the valve face of the specific gas cylinder for which the yoke was intended. This means that oxygen cylinders can only be connected to oxygen yokes as the pins of this yoke will only index or fit into the valve face of an oxygen cylinder (*Fig.* 3.16). Between the outlet orifice of the valve face and the yoke is a compressible rubber seal called a Bodok seal, without which the machine is unusable. Spare seals must therefore be available as they leak with prolonged use (*Fig.* 3.17).

Oxygen cylinders are coded black with a white cap and are filled to a pressure of about 1·2 MPa (1800 lbf/in^2 or 120 atm). As oxygen remains a gas at this pressure, the reading on the pressure gauge accurately reflects the cylinder content. Cylinders come in different sizes, the commonest

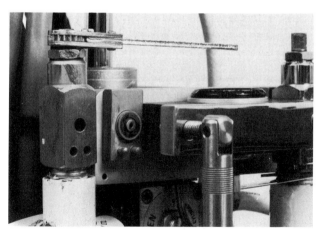

Fig. 3.16. The pins of an oxygen cylinder adjacent to the corresponding yoke fitting. The Bodok seal (*Fig.* 3.17) can be seen *in situ*.

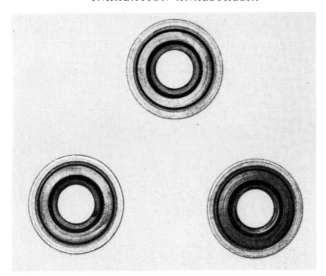

Fig. 3.17. Bodok seals. They comprise a compressible rubber seal surrounded by a narrow metal rim.

supplied for direct connection to an anaesthetic machine being size E, containing 24 cubic feet (680 litres) and size F, 48 cubic feet (1360 litres) of oxygen when full. With this knowledge it is possible to estimate the time that a full cylinder will supply a required flow rate from an anaesthetic machine.

Nitrous oxide cylinders are colour coded blue and as this agent is liquid at the pressure supplied, namely 5·2 MPa (750 lbf/in^2 or 50 atm) and 20 °C, the pressure inside will not be a reliable guide to the content as it will merely reflect the saturated vapour pressure of the liquid at this temperature. For this reason each cylinder is stamped with its tare (empty) weight and the nitrous oxide is sold by weight.

In some large hospitals the anaesthetic gases are supplied to the machine in pipelines which in turn are supplied from banks of very large cylinders with a reserve bank of cylinders onto which the supply is automatically switched when the pressure in the supply line falls to a predetermined value. Nevertheless, the anaesthetic machine must also carry its own spare cylinders of oxygen and nitrous oxide for use in case of a supply line failure.

The Anaesthetic Machine

Although there are various machines available today, they are all basic variations on the Boyle machine and have the following features in common (*Figs.* 3.18 and 3.19).

GENERAL ANAESTHESIA AND SEDATION IN DENTISTRY

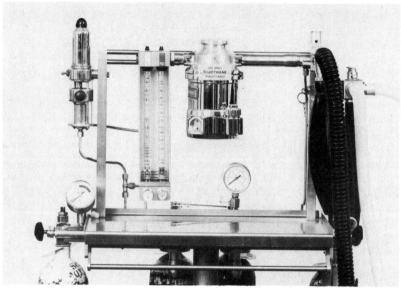

Fig. 3.18. A Boyle anaesthetic machine. Many variations are available but the standard features are shown in *Fig.* 3.19.

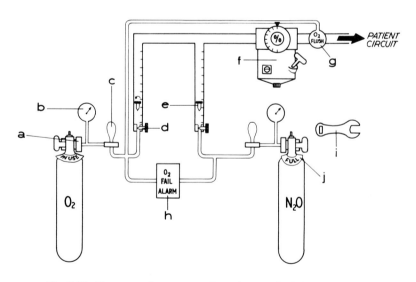

Fig. 3.19. Diagrammatic representation of a standard Boyle anaesthetic machine. The labelled features are discussed in the text.

INHALATION ANAESTHESIA

  a. A pair of yokes for both nitrous oxide and oxygen, i.e. one cylinder in use and one full spare cylinder ready for use.
  b. A pressure gauge to register the cylinder pressure at each yoke.
  c. A pressure reducing valve for each yoke. These valves serve two purposes. Firstly, they reduce the cylinder pressure from 120 atm (oxygen) or 50 atm (nitrous oxide) down to 4 atm (60 lbf/in^2) at which pressure the flow of gases can be controlled by the needle valves and visualized in the flow meters. Secondly, when an empty cylinder is removed from a yoke the replacement cylinder does not exhaust itself via the open yoke when it is opened, as the reducing valve acts as a one-way valve to isolate the yoke from atmosphere.
  d. Needle valves for each gas supplied, i.e. one for oxygen and one for nitrous oxide. These control the flow of gases through the rotameters.
  e. Rotameters which consist of tapered glass tubes containing bobbins which float and rotate in the gas stream. The rotameters are calibrated in flow rates of litres per minute marked on the walls of the glass tubes, and the reading is taken from the top of the bobbin. The bobbins must be seen to be rotating, as a non-rotating bobbin may be stuck against the wall of the tube and be giving a false reading.
  f. A calibrated vaporizer specific for the inhaled agent in use (either halothane or enflurane) which delivers a known concentration of the agent. In essence the vaporizer consists of a metal container placed in the line of flow of the anaesthetic gases. A sleeve valve splits the flow, sending a variable portion of the fresh gas flow through the part of the container containing the liquid to be vaporized (*Fig.* 3.20). This portion of the fresh

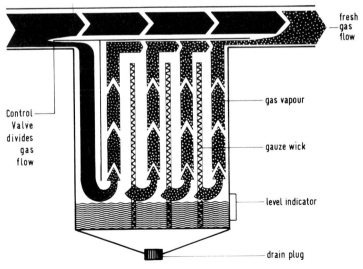

Fig. 3.20. Diagrammatic section of a calibrated vaporizer.

gas flow becomes saturated with the vapour of the liquid anaesthetic and is returned to the fresh gas flow which then continues into the anaesthetic circuit and on to the patient. Since, at constant temperature a known volume of fresh gas will be saturated with a constant percentage of vapour, the proportion of fresh gas passed through the vaporizer will determine the final percentage of vapour present in the inhaled mixture. In practice the temperature varies because the liquid anaesthetic cools as it is vaporized. However, modern vaporizers are temperature compensated to correct for the fall in vaporization with fall in temperature. Simple, non-temperature compensated vaporizers are still in use, for example, the Goldman dental vaporizer (*Fig.* 3.21). Their advantage lies in low cost and simplicity and they are satisfactory for repeated short cases. However, the percentage vapour falls with prolonged use as there is no temperature compensation.

g. In an emergency all anaesthetic machines must be capable of giving a 100% oxygen flush, i.e. a high flow rate of pure oxygen which by-passes the flow meter. This facility is clearly marked and controlled by a lever or knob marked 'emergency O_2'.

h. An oxygen failure alarm should be present to indicate failure of pressure in the oxygen supply line. This device can either be a whistle or siren driven by the pressure in the nitrous oxide line, or can be a battery operated device which flashes a warning light. As the alarm is activated before the needle valves and flow meters it will *not* warn of incorrect adjustment of the flow meter settings.

i. The spanner shown in the diagram is essential in that it fits the spindle valve shaft, and is therefore required to turn the cylinders on and off. Also the gland nut requires tightening as this sometimes allows gas to leak around the spindle itself. A spanner or ratchet *cylinder key* should be available for each set of cylinders.

j. Labels marking each cylinder of both nitrous oxide and oxygen either full or in use are essential and the labelling must be checked and confirmed at the start of each anaesthetic session as the cylinders labelled 'full' might not be so. Very occasionally it proves impossible to open the spindle valve on a full cylinder. Should the 'in use' cylinder run out during use the patient runs the risk of becoming hypoxic or waking up during the procedure.

Immediately prior to use, every anaesthetic machine must be checked to ensure that it is safe to use. The following points must be specifically noted. Both oxygen cylinders must have an appropriate content as judged by the pressures registered on the gauges. The cylinder marked 'full' must be so, and the 'in use' cylinder should be more than a quarter full. The oxygen cylinders should be changed before they empty completely as this will allow a margin of patient safety, should the valve on the full cylinder stick or fail to open. An empty cylinder must be changed immediately and

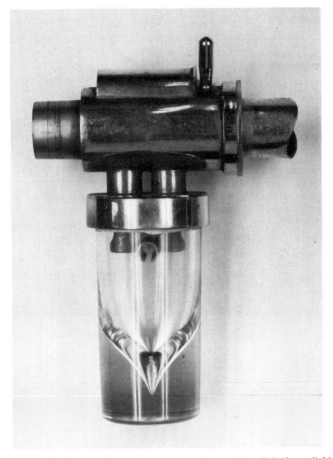

Fig. 3.21. The Goldman Vaporizer. It is the epitome of simplicity but reliable until the evaporation causes a fall in temperature thus reducing the percentage vaporization.

never be left on the machine. The emergency oxygen must also be tested and be seen to deliver an adequate oxygen flow rate into the patient circuit.

Although failure of the nitrous oxide supply may be embarrassing, it is never life threatening. Undetected failure of the oxygen supply in the machine is lethal. The oxygen failure alarm must be tested by switching off both oxygen cylinders, turning on the nitrous oxide cylinders and then turning on the oxygen flow meter. This bleeds the oxygen supply pressure in the machine to zero and should result in activation of the fail safe alarm. This test should be carried out before the patient is attached to the machine!

All the flow meter bobbins must be seen to be at the base of the flow meter tubes when the gas flows are turned off at the control needle valves, as bobbins sometimes stick at the top of the glass rotameter tube. Should a bobbin stick when in use an inappropriate gas flow may result.

The gas flow delivered by the machine should be tested by placing a thumb over the end of angle piece inside the face mask at the end of the patient circuit with an appropriate fresh gas flow set on the rotameter flow meters, the reservoir bag should be noted to fill and, with the expiratory valve fully closed, it should be possible to produce an adequate positive pressure against the thumb in the face mask by squeezing the reservoir bag.

Suitable Anaesthetic Circuits

There are essentially two circuits in use today:
1. The Magill circuit.
2. The Bain circuit.

These are illustrated in *Fig.* 3.22 and described below.

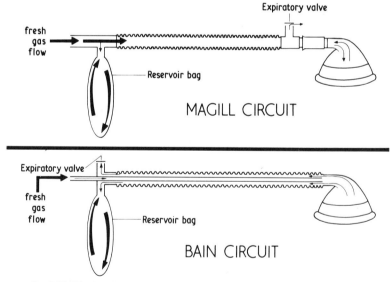

Fig. 3.22. The Magill and Bain circuits.

The Magill Circuit

The Magill circuit and its modifications, most widely used because of their simplicity and efficient use of the fresh gas flow, consist of a reservoir bag, supply tubing, mask and valve. Long use has led to an excellent understanding of its reliability and practicality. During inspiration the patient draws gas from the bag and the fresh gas flows via the tubing, the expiratory valve remains closed, and the bag partially collapses. During expiration the first increment of expired gas from the patient is dead space gas, i.e. its composition is the same as the fresh gas and it has not undergone respiratory exchange. This portion of the expired gas passes back into the tubing, as the fall in pressure in the tubing and bag brought about by inspiration is not reversed until the dead space gas is exhaled. When the combination of flow of fresh gas from the circuit plus the flow of exhaled gas from the patient is sufficient to fill the reservoir bag, the expiratory valve opens and the alveolar gas, i.e. that which has undergone respiratory exchange, passes out of the valve. In theory it is possible to adjust the fresh gas flow rate to equal the alveolar ventilation, i.e. 75% of the minute volume. A minor drawback of the standard Magill circuit is that scavenging of the exhaust gases from the expiratory valve tends to be cumbersome as this valve is situated on the mask end of the circuit. Modifications such as the Lack circuit appear to overcome this disadvantage by the use of co-axial tubing, but there are still some reservations concerning the resistance to expiration with this circuit.

The Bain Circuit

The Bain circuit is a more modern version of the T-piece, in essence a very simple circuit, but the elegant version of this co-axial circuit available commercially has led to its widespread use particularly for artificial ventilation. The internal continuity of the Bain circuit should be tested by filling the reservoir bag and then depressing the oxygen flush button, whereupon the bag will be seen to empty due to a Venturi effect. With spontaneous ventilation this circuit is very inefficient requiring a fresh gas flow of approximately $2\frac{1}{2}$ times the minute ventilation to avoid carbon dioxide retention. Although it is an easy circuit from which to scavenge waste gases its inefficiency limits its use in spontaneously breathing patients.

Anaesthetic machines and circuits designed for use in relative analgesia techniques are discussed in Chapter 4.

CHAPTER 4

INHALATION SEDATION (RELATIVE ANALGESIA)

Before discussing the particular concept of inhalation sedation the general nature of all sedation and its desirable qualities must be considered. The possibility of using drugs to affect patient attitudes to treatment, while maintaining a state of awareness, has been known and used for a long time; indeed the use of pure cocaine can fulfil this very purpose. The undesirable effects which may result cannot be overlooked, however, and the basis on which a sedative can be considered beneficial needs to be assessed. Such an agent would ideally:

1. Alleviate fear and anxiety.
2. Produce a degree of amnesia and analgesia.
3. Suppress vomiting reflexes but not protective reflexes.
4. Prolong potential operating time.
5. Be rapidly effective.
6. Have a sufficiently long effect which then quickly wears off.
7. Have no side-effects.
8. Be safely and easily administered by the operator.
9. Not require special procedures or precautions before or after use.

If the sedative agent fulfils the above requirements much general anaesthesia could be substituted by sedation. The uninterrupted use of nitrous oxide as the basic constituent of gaseous general anaesthetics demonstrates its acceptability and usefulness. Since the earliest days the amnesic and analgesic properties of the gas have been well known, but little was done to exploit these properties. The earliest use of nitrous oxide invariably relied upon a degree of anoxia to achieve anaesthesia since it is very difficult to achieve Stage III anaesthesia with concentrations of nitrous oxide below 80%. The first stage of anaesthesia, however, can often be achieved with concentrations as low as 20–25% of nitrous oxide and slightly higher dosage will certainly achieve its induction. This stage of amnesia and analgesia, accompanied by a degree of calmness, has been investigated and adopted by dental surgeons and obstetricians more than any other specialty of medicine and surgery under the name 'relative analgesia' (RA).

The effects of relative analgesia are primarily threefold:
1. There is a sedative effect.
2. There is an analgesic effect.
3. There is a degree of anterograde amnesia.

Additionally there is some suppression of all reflexes and a general slowing of responses but the coughing mechanism appears to be minimally affected. Vomiting is rare but very occasionally seen, the incidence

INHALATION SEDATION (RELATIVE ANALGESIA)

being under 1%. The various psychomotor and sensory effects of RA are illustrated in *Fig.* 4.1. It can be seen that three overlapping planes of analgesia are recognized and that the effects tend to be somewhat variable within each plane. The most desirable state of analgesia is in the border region between planes I and II, normally requiring a 20% nitrous oxide

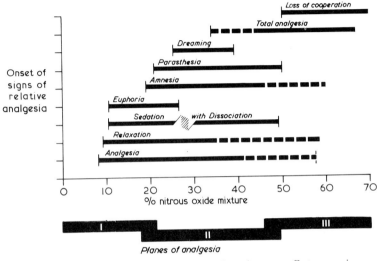

Fig. 4.1. Diagram to illustrate the sensory and psychomotor effects occurring during stage I anaesthesia, (stage of analgesia) (*see also Fig.* 3.1).

content. The duration of the action of nitrous oxide can be controlled and the very quick clearance time has already been discussed in Chapter 2.

It should be noted that none of the attributes of RA should be considered total. The depth of sedation and analgesia can vary quite considerably from patient to patient and even on different occasions. The degree of amnesia may also vary but usually to a lesser degree. It is these potential variations which constitute the only serious problem in using nitrous oxide as a sedative. The fact that an intravenous injection is not required and the safety of RA constitute important benefits in its favour.

The safety aspect derives principally from the level of anaesthesia which can be achieved with the standard RA machines. The details of these are described later but their design incorporates devices which prevent the volume ratio of the nitrous oxide/oxygen mixture being greater than 77/23%. The *theoretical* maximum concentration of nitrous oxide obtainable in a circuit is 77% but in practice it is often lower since a leak-free circuit is virtually unobtainable. This is due to the movements of the patient and the work of the dental surgeon breaking the seal of the mask.

In addition to the machine safety factor, the maximum benefit from the amnesic, sedative and analgesic properties comes in the middle part of Stage I anaesthesia and any deepening into Stage II will produce excitement and an increased response to painful stimuli. This is fairly easily prevented by never allowing the nitrous oxide level to rise over 50% and by carefully monitoring patient's responses to produce the correct level of sedation. Many operators fail to realize the undesirable effects of this fact and automatically start patients on high nitrous oxide concentrations. It is of little surprise that their success rate tends to be higher with intravenous agents where an increased dosage will result in deeper sedation. Initial reaction to a developing lack of co-operation should therefore be to reduce the plane of analgesia by reducing the nitrous oxide flow, or, if low volumes of gas are being administered, increasing the oxygen flow.

The third advantage of nitrous oxide in relative analgesia is its safety as a drug. There is minimal disturbance of the protective reflexes and because of its low solubility in the blood it is quickly cleared from the blood stream in the lungs, within 5 min of breathing normal air. Very occasionally patients are encountered who are exceptionally sensitive to nitrous oxide and who, even with concentrations below 50%, become anaesthetized. It is essential that the high safety factor of nitrous oxide does not become an excuse for casualness and lack of care, but rather it should be seen as allowing one the opportunity to develop and perfect a useful technique.

RELATIVE ANALGESIA EQUIPMENT

Machines specifically designed for nitrous oxide sedation as opposed to anaesthesia have been developed over the past 30 years in both Germany and America. In Britain their history is more recent and aspects of their structure are continually being refined. Currently virtually all machines in use are of the continuous-flow type and the old demand-flow machines are becoming obsolete.

Two types of machine are in common use in the United Kingdom. Their features both include:-

1. Minimum oxygen delivery of 30% gas volume.
2. Emergency oxygen over-ride at over 10 litres/min.
3. Automatic cut-out if oxygen delivery falls below 30%.
4. Visual flowmeters. (These operate on a slightly different principle from the rotameters described in Chapter 3. They consist of a weighted ball bearing which is propelled up a sloping calibrated tube by the gas flow. Readings are then taken from the centre of the bearing.)
5. Reservoir bag and control valves to allow manual ventilation in emergency.

The main variation between the machines (*Figs.* 4.2 and 4.3) are that the Quantiflex Marks I and II deliver 3 litres oxygen per minute as soon as

INHALATION SEDATION (RELATIVE ANALGESIA)

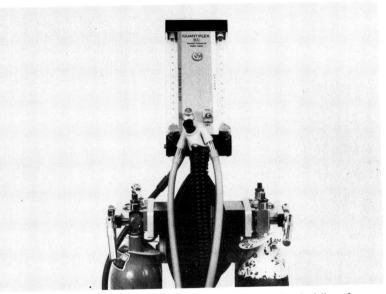

Fig. 4.2. The Quantiflex (Mark I). When switched on it immediately delivers 3 litres/min oxygen, (the Mark II is similar).

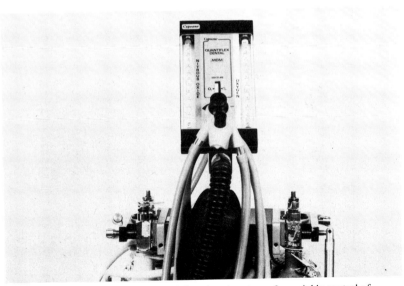

Fig. 4.3. The MDM Quantiflex. It has the advantage of a variable control of the actual gas volume delivered thus saving awkward calculations should the minute volumes need altering.

GENERAL ANAESTHESIA AND SEDATION IN DENTISTRY

they are switched on. The MDM Quantiflex allows a variable percentage of the delivered (and also variable) minute volume. This is less wasteful of the gases and allows easier control of the relative gas proportions without necessarily having to vary the minute volume. Both types of machine have nasal masks with 'air-mixer valves'. These allow dilution of the gas mixture with air but in a manner which cannot be controlled and for this reason are not very satisfactory. It is also a cause of air pollution which until recently has been a problem with RA. A customized expiratory circuit is available which attaches to the nosepiece and removes excess or expired gases (*Fig.* 4.4).

The apparatus should always be checked before use. Each gas cylinder should be individually turned on, and the pressure dial checked. The

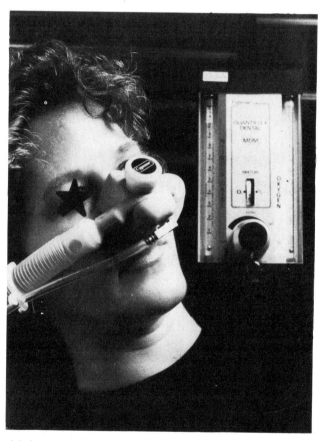

Fig. 4.4. A customized expiratory circuit. It can operate passively or actively (or both).

maximum flow of gas should then be operated and the dial rechecked to ensure that there is no decrease in pressure. If such a decrease occurs it signifies that either the gas cylinder is low or that there is obstruction in the early (high pressure) part of the circuit. The nosepiece should then be occluded with a hand to check the patency of the expiratory valve. The valve should then be closed and the bag allowed to inflate before it is squeezed hard. The gases should be forced past the hand occluding the mask or a leak is indicated. The effectiveness of the safety valve which should cut the nitrous oxide off in the event of oxygen failure can be checked by running the gases together at 5 l/min each. The oxygen cylinder is then turned off and the nitrous oxide should cut-out immediately the flow of oxygen reduces to 3 l/min. It is this safety mechanism that makes this technique so acceptable for use by an operator/administrator but it is very prudent to check that it is functioning each time the machine is used. It is important that the valves are released before proceeding with the sedation technique.

PREPARING PATIENTS FOR RELATIVE ANALGESIA

Because of the nature of its action and its easy administration, RA is particularly suitable for use in nervous children who have a basic desire and will to be co-operative. A state of ataraxia (peacefulness) is required and there is little doubt that this is achieved by a combination of suggestion and semi-hypnosis, and is not solely the result of the nitrous oxide.

Patients with severe respiratory disease can present an increased risk. In particular, patients with chronic bronchitis or emphysema should not be treated as the higher-than-air oxygen content of the mixture can abolish their drive to breathe. Psychiatrically disturbed patients are best treated in hospital. RA is particularly suitable in apprehensive or fearful children, particularly those who are phobic about injections. Similarly adults with 'needle phobia' and those who find dental treatment stressful may respond well to RA. The relaxation produced can also be used to good effect in treating hyperactive or physically handicapped patients.

Suitably selected patients should be given the same instructions as for a general anaesthetic with the exception that light snacks are permissible 2–3 h preoperatively. If there is any possibility that the work may have to be completed under general anaesthesia, however, patients should adhere to the full instructions including 6 h starvation. The patients should be informed before their visit that they will not be going right off to sleep and they should be re-informed of this fact before proceeding with sedation. Patients who understand what is about to happen to them, approach their appointment in a calmer and more relaxed manner than a nervous patient who is unsure of the procedure. In consequence their respiration is more regular and induction of RA can proceed in a smooth and steady fashion.

The need for co-operation cannot be stressed enough since the very nature of its continuous administration requires uninterrupted patient co-operation. It has been suggested that the need for patient–operator interaction makes RA more akin to hypnosis than it does to other types of sedation. Whilst this may or may not be true, there is little doubt that successful RA is only achieved with frequent reassurance and encouragement.

ADMINISTERING RELATIVE ANALGESIA

The apparatus having been checked and the patient instructed in what is to happen, the induction can now proceed. The supine position is without doubt the most suitable position for RA both from the technical and physiological viewpoints. It will minimize the chances of fainting and allows easier access to the mouth as the nosepiece more easily sits in position. Patients who complain of discomfort can be treated in the modified Trendelenburg position, (*Fig.* 4.5). People with a history of

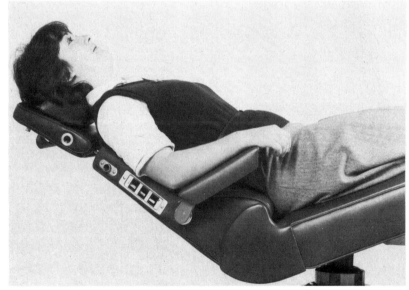

Fig. 4.5 The Trendelenburg position involves the feet being raised to a higher level than the head. In the dental chair it is achieved by laying back the patient and then tilting the chair. The modified position (shown) uses full tilt but only partial lie-back.

cardiac problems, complaining of chest pain or dyspnoea, are more safely postponed at this stage and referred for a consultant opinion. (Patients with such problems are occasionally treated with RA in hospital. The sitting position is adopted as it lowers the venous return and consequently reduces the cardiac output.)

The patient is told in detail what is proposed and shown the various parts of the machine, in particular the nosepiece. The need for a personal approach must be re-emphasized since this is a technique requiring patient co-operation, which is more easily achieved when they are fully aware of what is about to happen. The machine should then be switched on and the oxygen level increased to about 5 l/min. The patency of the expiratory valve is rechecked and the mask gently applied to the patient, telling them that only pure oxygen is being administered and that they will feel no effects yet. Slow regular breathing is essential and patients should be encouraged to do this before proceeding with the administration of nitrous oxide. Occasionally patients have untoward reactions at this stage and if gentle reassurance cannot calm them it is unlikely that the nitrous oxide sedation will have much effect, and it is wise to discontinue the technique.

Table 4.1. Relative Flow Rates for Varying N_2O/O_2 Ratios

Total flow rate (litres/min)	Flow rate (litres/min)									
	N_2O 10%	O_2 90%	N_2O 20%	O_2 80%	N_2O 30%	O_2 70%	N_2O 40%	O_2 60%	N_2O 50%	O_2 50%
3	0·3	2·7	0·6	2·4	0·9	2·1	1·2	1·8	1·5	1·5
4	0·4	3·6	0·8	3·2	1·2	2·8	1·6	2·4	2	2
5	0·5	4·5	1·0	4·0	1·5	3·5	2·0	3·0	2·5	2·5
6	0·6	5·4	1·2	4·8	1·8	4·2	2·4	3·6	3	3
7	0·7	6·3	1·4	5·6	2·1	4·9	2·8	4·2	3·5	3·5
8	0·8	7·2	1·6	6·4	2·4	5·6	3·2	4·8	4	4
9	0·9	8·1	1·8	7·2	2·7	6·3	3·6	5·4	4·5	4·5

The various percentage gas flows at any given volume per min. The shaded boxes do not apply as the Quantiflex Mark I does not operate below 3 litres O_2 per min.

Assuming all is proceeding uneventfully, the nitrous oxide flow can be slowly introduced and increased over a period of 2–3 min. The concentration of nitrous oxide can of course be varied by changing the flow of either gas and a table of the relative percentage flows related to the volume of the gas flows is shown in *Table* 4.1. On the MDM Quantiflex this is obviously much simpler.

The actual percentages of gases being administered should be titrated against the patient's response. At all stages the patient should respond to speech although at times the response may be a little slow. The effects of nitrous oxide vary, the more obvious being a warm sensation, a feeling of relaxation and general well being. Less desirably but frequently present are a tingling feeling in the toes, fingers or lips, a dizzy light-headed (floating) sensation and occasionally the famous 'giggles' for which nitrous oxide (laughing) gas is so well known (*Fig.* 4.6).

Continuous conversation should be maintained with the patient while carefully observing the signs of satisfactory analgesia. The occurrence of each sign is, however, unreliable and the sedative, analgesic and amnesic effects are obviously the most useful and significant. Fortunately, the less

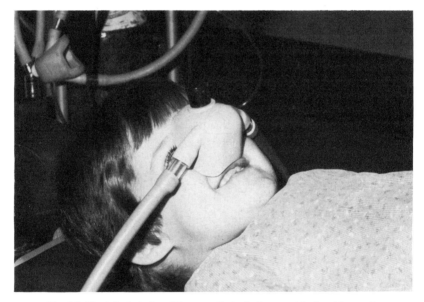

Fig. 4.6. The 'giggles'. A well-known effect of nitrous oxide (laughing gas).

desirable effects are seen most commonly in the deeper end of Stage I and reducing the nitrous oxide/oxygen ratio will often reverse them. This is contrary to the actions taken by many operators since they feel that because of the disturbances, deeper sedation is needed. While in one sense they are correct, it is certainly not achieved by increasing the nitrous oxide/oxygen ratio as this only results in an increased likelihood of Stage II anaesthesia (with all its consequent problems). The process of induction should take several minutes, particularly on the first occasion. It is acceptable on subsequent visits to rapidly induce analgesia by increasing the nitrous oxide ratio to the predetermined level within seconds of commencing.

When the patient is settled the volumes of gas flowing can be noted for reference on future occasions. During quiet respiration the valve should be observed between expiration and inspiration. If there is much loss of gases the overall flow should be reduced while maintaining the same gas/oxygen ratio. On the other hand if there is no noise and the patient appears to be making increased respiratory effort the volumes should be increased, again maintaining the same ratio. On average the healthy adult has a minute volume of 5 l/min. The tidal volumes of children are smaller but the respiratory rate may be quicker so the minute volume is not directly proportional to size and should be estimated from patient to patient.

During RA it is essential to maintain verbal contact with the patient by giving occasional instructions and checking they are obeyed. Although the use of mouth props can make treatment easier they must be avoided since they may decrease the operator's awareness as to the state of his patient. Occasionally patients themselves wish to lighten the plane of sedation and they should be instructed how to do this by mouth breathing. Excess gases will then be lost through the expiratory valve or taken up in the scavenger circuit. Recurrent mouth breathing should indicate to the operator that the nitrous oxide/oxygen ratio is too high or that insufficient gases are flowing and the patient is finding nose breathing uncomfortable. Alternatively some patients wish to experience greater effects and by taking deeper breaths they may obtain slight increase in the depth of analgesia. Care should be taken before increasing the nitrous oxide/oxygen ratio and signs of disturbance should usually indicate the need for its reduction.

There is a need for local anaesthesia to supplement RA in all but the most basic of procedures, particularly with adult patients. Local anaesthesia is usually well tolerated, the pain threshold having been raised and sensation awareness of the needle being much duller than normal. Conservative or surgical procedures can then be accomplished with little disturbance. On completion the patient is informed that treatment is over and that they must breathe oxygen for a couple of minutes. The nitrous oxide will actually clear slightly quicker from the blood if normal air is breathed since the high oxygen content has a small depressing effect on the respiratory drive. However, it is easier to monitor the patients' recovery while they lie still and so most operators adopt the plan of running 100% oxygen for 2 min. This method also minimizes the remote possibility of nitrous oxide hypoxia explained in Chapter 2. Within 10 min the patient should be clear headed and the nitrous oxide virtually cleared from the blood. Although there should be no theoretical objection to patients driving away, it is not permissible for medico-legal reasons.

The use of RA gives an excellent type of sedation in well selected patients. Particularly suitable are children, co-operative but anxious patients, and those with medical ailments which could make general anaesthesia a risk. Supportive treatment for anxious patients, using a technique with a safety margin as high as RA obviously deserves greater emphasis and its benefits need promoting. It is also a useful technique to use in early treatment planning with a view to gradually weaning the patient away from sedation. There are, however, still patients in whom the effects of RA are not satisfactory and there still remains a place for the use of oral and intravenous sedation.

CHAPTER 5

INTRAVENOUS ANAESTHESIA

The development of intravenous anaesthetics can in some ways be traced back to the seventeenth century when Sir Christopher Wren experimented with injections of opium and alcoholic drinks (usually rum or beer). These were given to dogs using a sharpened quill with a reservoir. He noted that with lower doses the animals recovered and at higher doses they died. In a sense he discovered what is the fundamental difference between intravenous and inhalational anaesthesia, that is once a substance has been injected it cannot be removed. Despite this limitation, however, the use of intravenous techniques has multiplied over the past 40 years when previously only inhalational methods would have been used.

The basic indications for general anaesthesia were considered in Chapter 1. The specific indications for using intravenous agents include:
1. A quick induction is required.
2. A very short anaesthetic is predicted.
3. The patient fears masks.
4. The desire to avoid halogenated vapours.
5. Intubation is anticipated.
6. Incremental techniques are to be used.

The agents and the technique should also be well suited and would be:
1. Capable of easy administration.
2. Free from side- or after-effects.
3. Quickly effective and predictable in duration.
4. Have a wide safety margin.
5. Allow rapid return of any lost reflexes.
6. Quickly excreted or metabolized.
7. Stable in aqueous solution and have a long shelf-life.
8. Non-toxic to local tissues.

The factors that are potentially variable in terms of ease of administration are the volume required to give a therapeutic dose and the viscosity of the fluid. Low and high volumes both have disadvantages, the former due to the need for extra care in controlling the injection and the latter in terms of the time it takes to complete. Time is also a problem with excessively viscous agents since they must be injected slowly to avoid thrombotic or embolic effects.

The acceptability, or not, of side- and after-effects is to some extent a matter of personal decision. Those agents which affect the medullary centre in normal doses are unacceptable since the disturbance of respiratory or cardiovascular physiology is potentially lethal. Similarly while after-effects of nausea and headache may be commonly accepted by patients, they should obviously be avoided if possible.

Most modern agents are quickly effective and while variation in effective times does occur, it is usually only within certain acceptable limits (a few seconds). Recovery times are usually related to the speed of redistribution rather than excretory or metabolic action. Because of this repeated or incremental doses must be much reduced in terms of their dosage as a baseline blood level remains and the speed of redistribution decreases. The actual safety margin of a drug can be estimated by comparing an average lethal dose (LD50) with the average therapeutic dose (TD50). The ratio LD50/TD50 is often referred to as the therapeutic ratio or index; the higher the ratio the safer the drug, particularly when one considers that the dose given has to be based on such factors as weight, metabolic rate, emotional state, age and medical history, etc. The speed of recovery is dependent on several factors. As stated most drugs will be redistributed, thus the plasma concentration falls (*Fig.* 5.1). It is

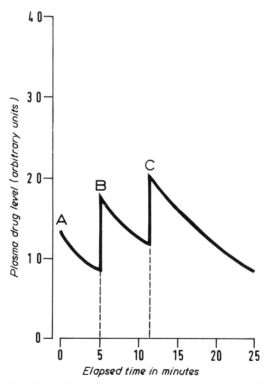

Fig. 5.1. The effects of multiple injection of a hypothetical drug. The rate of decay and the peaks of plasma concentration are mainly affected by the half-life of the drug, which in the example given is about 11–12 min.

usually then metabolized and excreted over the next 12–48 h. Any decrease in the speed of redistribution or any increase in the total administered dose will reduce the rate of recovery, this being in addition to the patient's own sensitivity to the drug. This slowish clearance also means that if another dose of the agent is given within the period of metabolism, the patient will exhibit increased sensitivity. The authors have seen cases of respiratory and circulatory collapse following repeated administration when this factor was not taken into account. Before examining the clinical attributes of the various agents and methods it is essential that a sound venepuncture technique is established.

VENEPUNCTURE

It has been said that venepuncture is 90% preparation and 10% injection and while the figures may be arbitrary there is much in the spirit of this statement. The basis for sound venepuncture is a good knowledge of anatomy and skilful technique. Two sites have been commonly used:

1. The ante-cubital fossa—ideal because of its large veins and stability regardless of hand movements.
2. The back of the hand—useful if a needle is to be left *in situ* as it is less likely to displace into the tissues.

The anatomy of these sites is shown in *Figs.* 5.2 and 5.3.

Before proceeding further the anaesthetist should check that all the required equipment is at hand and working, both for the venepuncture and for subsequent anaesthesia. The supine or modified Trendelenburg position is preferred though some anaesthetists still prefer the sitting (upright) position.

The anticipated volume of the agent, plus a little extra, should be drawn into a syringe using a large bore needle. This will help to avoid excessive air in the solution. The syringe can then be tapped repeatedly to displace air inclusions before attaching a small gauge needle. Small needles are less painful to use and easier to insert, but may prove difficult to use with viscous agents. Syringes over 5 ml in size should have eccentric hubs so the needle can be kept parallel with the skin after insertion. Otherwise manually bending the needle is an acceptable alternative.

The vein to be used should be prepared to provide maximum dilatation. Veins can be extremely difficult to visualize or palpate in obese patients, cold or nervous individuals or in those who have had repeated venepunctures for one reason or another. This can be improved by warming the skin and with repeated light tapping. Maximum dilatation of the vein is obtained if a cuff is pressurized midway between diastolic and systolic pressure, since this allows maximal filling with minimal drainage. In difficult patients it is often worth using a sphygmomanometer to achieve this. Usually it is satisfactory to use one of the proprietary elasticated cuffs

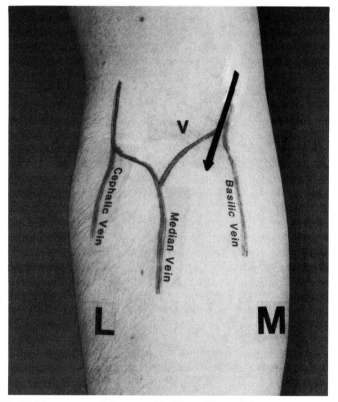

Fig. 5.2. The anatomy of the ante-cubital fossa. The medial (M) and lateral (L) aspects of the arm are marked and the V represents the insertion of the biceps tendon. The black arrow indicates the path of the brachial artery near which is the median nerve (not shown). Where the median vein diverges it forms the median-cephalic vein and median-basilic veins respectively.

tightened so as to allow the passage of arterial blood into the arm, but sufficient to occlude the venous return. Repeated clenching of the fist also helps to improve the venous return.

Once the vein is palpable the skin may be cleansed with an antiseptic swab containing isopropyl alcohol. The skin is then tensed with the left hand and the syringe held as shown in *Fig.* 5.4. The syringe barrel should be held 'overhand' and no attempt made to hold below the barrel, which would obstruct venepuncture.

The needle is first inserted quickly into the subcutaneous tissues before being advanced at a slightly steeper angle until the vein is punctured. With experience this is detectable by a sudden decrease in the resistance to the

INTRAVENOUS ANAESTHESIA

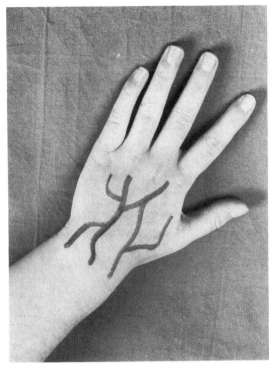

Fig. 5.3. The superficial veins of the hand. Individual variation is marked but two or three good veins running longitudinally can usually be visualized.

needle. Successful venepunctures should be demonstrated by positive aspiration of blood of the correct colour; the cuff is then released and the injection can proceed.

The use of the ante-cubital fossa is extremely popular but it does present certain hazards. The brachial artery and median nerve both run in a fairly superficial position on the medial aspect of the arm. The insertion of the biceps tendon acts as a very good landmark on which to base the anatomical geography of the fossa since injections given laterally to the tendon are safe and those given medially carry substantially greater risk.

Other aspects of venepuncture tend to be controversial. The authors prefer the bevel of the needle upwards so that the vein can be lifted during the injection, thus enabling some visualization of the injection. Some would argue that the bevel downwards is less likely to result in the needle penetrating the deeper wall of the vein and 'tissuing', which gives a characteristic bubbling of the skin. The use of topical anaesthetics is seldom necessary despite those who advocate its wholesale use.

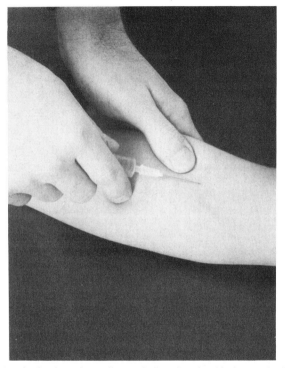

Fig. 5.4. Injection into the median-cephalic vein. The skin is tensed with the thumb of the left hand and the syringe is held overhand. (It can only be gripped round the barrel by bending the needle.)

Once an injection has been completed the needle should be withdrawn quickly and smoothly. Firm pressure is then applied with a gauze swab and a proprietary dressing applied if necessary. If repeated injections are thought likely, the needle should be secured with sticky tapes after its initial insertion. Usually in such cases the butterfly needle is more useful and this is probably best inserted into the back of the hand (*Fig.* 5.5). These types of needles are most easily inserted into a vein which has just united from two smaller vessels, or into a large straight vein.

The complications of venepuncture include erroneous intra-arterial injection, injection into the median nerve in the ante-cubital fossa or venous thrombosis. These are dealt with in Chapter 8. Having successfully punctured a vein and administered an agent, there are broadly three possibilities:
  1. Complete the treatment on the induction dose.
  2. Use an incremental technique (repeat administration).
  3. Proceed to an inhalational anaesthetic (Chapters 3 and 7).

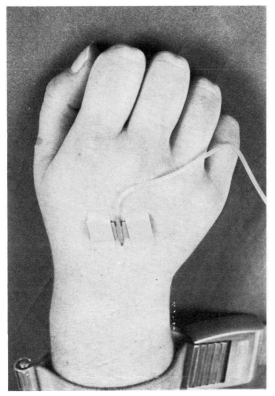

Fig. 5.5. A butterfly needle *in situ*. It should be taped as shown but in practice it is more easily taped across the wings.

Successfully completing treatment on a single dose of short-acting intravenous anaesthetic is not easy. It should only be attempted by a team of a competent operator and anaesthetist. Patients seldom lose their muscle tone and so opening the mouth is particularly difficult. To facilitate this, a mouth prop can be placed in position just before venepuncture or even as the injection is being given. Once inserted the jaw should be supported by an assistant as patients find props extremely uncomfortable to keep in place even for short periods. The anaesthetist should then devote all his attention to maintaining the airway so that respiratory function is not compromised. Short periods of respiratory depression following intravenous induction can quickly result in cyanosis, particularly as the atmosphere contains less oxygen than the gas mixtures normally used in inhalational anaesthetics.

The second technique mentioned involves repeated injections of the agent. The method depends on the redistribution of the anaesthetic as

described in Chapter 2. Small increments (usually 20–30% of the original dose) are administered when the patient shows signs of wakening, i.e. making spontaneous noise or movements. The plasma concentration is then raised to at least its former level and declines at a slower rate to the level at which consciousness will return. There are one or two problems with this technique:
1. The incremental dose and requirements are somewhat arbitrary.
2. Prolonged recovery is progressively more likely.
3. Overdosage is likely.
4. No analgesia is normally provided by the anaesthetic.
5. Problems of airway obstruction can be acute.

Even so incremental methods do have their place in modern dentistry, but not with the operator/anaesthetist. The operator/anaesthetist is unacceptable since it has been shown that however light one tries to maintain an anaesthetic, some patients will fail to protect their own airway. This technique is therefore only suitable when administered by a trained anaesthetist, who can give the agents, whilst continually observing the airway.

The third use of intravenous agents is as a precursor to inhalational anaesthesia. It is useful in that:
1. It avoids patient awareness of the mask and gases.
2. It leads to rapid loss of consciousness.
3. It avoids Stage II of anaesthesia.
4. It allows greater control of the airway.

These reasons tend to make it popular for use in adult patients. The disadvantages are:
1. It is difficult in those who are phobic about needles.
2. It occasionally results in apnoea or hiccuping.
3. There is no leeway for error in that Stage II may not be completed, during the gas administration and the concurrent fall in plasma concentration of the intravenous agent.

For inpatient anaesthesia these difficulties can be eased by premedicating the patient. This technique is by far the most common to be used preceeding intubation. In the outpatient situation premedication is not usually possible and complications must be dealt with as they arise. Such complications are relatively few, however, and the drugs in modern usage are, on the whole, extremely safe. The clinical nature of some of the popular drugs in current use are considered below, the pharmacological aspects of these agents having been considered in Chapter 2.

Methohexitone

Methohexitone is an ultra-short acting water-soluble methyl-barbiturate. It is by far the most popular agent used in intravenous practice. Its advantages are several.

INTRAVENOUS ANAESTHESIA

1. It is short-acting but predictable.
2. It is potent.
3. It allows early postoperative ambulation.
4. It can be used incrementally.
5. It has a relatively low tissue toxicity.
6. It is metabolized relatively quickly—its half-life usually being under 2 h.

The problems which can arise with methohexitone are:

1. Hiccuping (or coughing).
2. Extraneous (epileptiform) muscle activity.
3. Pain on injection.

It has been said for these reasons that methohexitone should not be used on epileptic patients, but there is no evidence in the literature to provide any direct relationship.

Methohexitone induces sleep in one arm-to-brain circulation time (18–25 s) and is effective for 3–7 min in basic therapeutic dosage. There can be little doubt that its advantages outweigh its disadvantages and that this accounts for its marked popularity. It is injected in a dose of 1·0–1·5 mg/kg of body weight in adults in either a 1% or 2% solution. Slightly higher doses are required in children.

Thiopentone

Thiopentone is the most popularly used intravenous anaesthetic in the world and is to some extent the basic agent against which all others are compared. It is a water-soluble, rapidly acting member of the thiobarbiturates. It produces a smooth induction usually free of extraneous muscle activity. Its other advantages include:

1. Predictable action.
2. Potent.
3. Suitable for incremental use—but only in short procedures.
4. Minimal side-effects.

It does have disadvantages which make it less suitable for outpatient use:

1. Slower recovery.
2. Relatively tissue toxic due mainly to a high pH.
3. It is unstable in aqueous solution despite its easy solubility.
4. Patients may respond unpredictably to painful stimuli.
5. In higher doses it may lead to respiratory and cardiovascular depression.

It is these factors which have precluded thiopentone from taking the leading position in outpatient dentistry. It is redistributed quickly following injection being effective from 4 to 12 min. It is metabolized much more slowly than methohexitone.

Barbiturates are known to potentiate alcohol and certain sedatives, so the longer metabolites or the unmetabolized drug remain in the blood, the longer a patient needs to take precautions.

Thiopentone is only about 40% as potent as methohexitone. It is usually therefore given in 2·5% aqueous solution, made freshly for each session. The dosage can be calculated approximately from the weight of the patient, being between 2·5 and 5 mg/kg of body weight. A maximum dose of 500 mg need seldom be exceeded though allowances may have to be made for those who receive regular sedatives, drink excessively or who are extremely large. Conversely, there are occasions when the medical history renders a smaller dose more appropriate.

Althesin

Althesin is a mixture of two quick-acting steroid anaesthetics (alphaxalone and alphadolone) dissolved in Cremophor, which is derived from castor oil. It is not water soluble but has found a leading place in anaesthesia due primarily to its smooth, if slightly slow, action and its extremely high therapeutic index, which is nearly five times that of thiopentone and methohexitone. Unfortunately, it has been reported on several occasions as giving rise to acute sensitivity reactions of the anaphylactic type. If patients with allergic histories of any type are avoided it is probably the anaesthetic agent of choice for inducing high risk patients. Its favourable properties may be summarized as:

1. Safe, good quality anaesthesia.
2. Minimal cardiovascular or respiratory side-effects.
3. Predictable duration of anaesthesia.
4. Rapid recovery (between methohexitone and thiopentone).
5. Hangover and postoperative sickness rare.
6. Suitable for intermittent injection for moderate periods of time.

Its side-effects include:

1. Risk of hypersensitivity (at least 10 times greater than barbiturates).
2. Extraneous movements may occur (tremulous rather than epileptiform).
3. Not suitable for use in patients with porphyria (i.e. it is not a feasible alternative to barbiturates which should also be avoided).

Of these side-effects the first is the only real problem. It should be pointed out that the reactions encountered are almost all due to the solvent Cremophor which has also been reported as causing similar incidents when used independently from Althesin. Thus it would appear that if the drug companies could produce a water soluble steroid type anaesthetic of otherwise similar qualities, it would represent a potential advance in the available agents. Since it is a mixture of two drugs, its dose is measured in millilitres, an average adult dose being up to 5 ml.

Etomidate

Etomidate is presently the most modern commercially available agent marketed in the United Kingdom. It is fundamentally different from all the other agents discussed being a complex dextro-isomer of an organic carboxylate sulphate. The white crystals of etomidate are highly soluble in water but tend to be unstable once prepared so it is prepared commercially pre-dissolved in an organic solvent containing 35% propylene glycol.

It is effective in an average time of about 10 s, but individual variation can be between 5 and 25 s. Broadly speaking, it has the same induction properties as methohexitone.

Thereafter, it appears that there is an initial redistribution followed by rapid metabolism. This is due to the effect of hepatic and plasma esterases causing hydrolysis of the drug. It is said to have minimal cardiovascular effects and indeed has a high therapeutic index—three times that of methohexitone.

It is not the perfect agent, however, and there are disadvantages. The most obvious of these is the relatively high number of patients who exhibit extraneous movements. Occasionally, this develops into a hypertonic state which makes dental treatment extremely difficult. The cause of this is unclear and it may be due to the pain frequently experienced during injection. Using large veins and slower injections gives the clinical impression of a lower incidence of induction upsets. It can also be reduced by using a narcotic type of premedication, which would make it unsuitable for outpatient anaesthesia. Thus, one may summarize its advantages as:

1. Safe, modern anaesthetic.
2. Minimal cardiovascular depression.
3. Predictable duration of anaesthesia.
4. Rapid smooth recovery.
5. Quickly effective.

Its disadvantages may be summarized as:

1. Frequently produces painful injection.
2. Extraneous muscular activity common.
3. Causes hiccuping (less than methohexitone).
4. Postoperative vomiting more common than with barbiturates.

The use of etomidate will probably increase though the extent of its full acceptance is difficult to predict. It has been tried as an incremental anaesthetic with some success and as a sedative with limited success. It is not the ideal induction agent and the quality of anaesthesia while acceptable is not as high as that of Althesin. A weight related dose of 0·3 mg/kg body weight is standard.

Propanidid

This agent has been in use for nearly 40 years and is a derivative of eugenol. It is not commonly used but it is nonetheless an interesting and useful drug in certain circumstances. Its main feature is the extremely rapid and complete recovery which it exhibits, due not to its redistribution, but to its metabolism by plasma cholinesterase. This reduces it to a metabolite with no anaesthetic properties at all.

After injection rapid loss of consciousness is followed immediately by a short period of hyperventilation (this can be so marked that experts in blind nasal intubation have used the inspiratory phase to pass an endotracheal tube). Loss of consciousness varies from 1 to 5 min and recovery is usually smooth. Unfortunately, a few anaphylactic reactions have been reported and while this is probably due to the solvent (Cremophor) for this and other reasons propanidid is not widely used. Its rapid metabolism makes it suitable for dental work, which can be completed very quickly, but it is not a drug which is of use in incremental techniques. An adult dose of 5–7 mg/kg body weight is normal and the drug is supplied in 500-mg ampoules of 10 ml.

Ketamine

This is an agent of such a different nature that its use is confined to extremely specific situations, all inpatient. It is a water soluble derivative of the phencyclidine group. Its biggest advantage is that it can be injected intramuscularly if required. Unfortunately, however, it is slow to take effect, often results in hypertonus and occasionally fairly marked hypertension. Its most unfortunate side-effects, being particularly common in adults, are vivid hallucinations, awakening delirium and tunnel vision, all of which may last for periods up to 24 h.

There is no doubt that these side-effects can be reduced markedly by using opiate or diazepam (or both) premedication. Additionally, low concentrations of halothane help to stabilize the blood pressure assuming its use is acceptable. If the blood pressure rises markedly a combined α, β blocking agent such as labetalol should be given.

It is clear that this is not a drug for outpatient use but one which may be suitable for certain specific or difficult situations.

PRACTICAL OUTPATIENT TECHNIQUES

The inherent safety of a carefully given intravenous anaesthetic cannot be disputed since vast numbers are given each year in outpatient situations with very few incidents. This is due to:
1. Careful selection of patients.
2. Familiarity with techniques.
3. The safe nature of most agents.
4. The self-protection of the patient even during anaesthesia.

INTRAVENOUS ANAESTHESIA

To ensure the first two points is essential: to depend on the second two is folly. The selection of patients was discussed in Chapter 1 and points 3 and 4 above have been elaborated in this and previous chapters. Familiarity with techniques can only be gained by practical experience, and while some of the hazards are discussed below, there is no substitute for clinical experience in dealing with the various mishaps which may occur. Several problems are encountered during intravenous anaesthesia which differ from those of inhalational anaesthesia.

Assessing Doses

Most drugs are supplied with guide dose charts, but the individual variation can be extreme. The arm-to-brain circulation time means a delay of up to 30 s before one can assess the effects of an injected dose. In doing this the loss of muscle tone and the strength or lack of the eyelash reflex should be noted. If, after half a minute they have not reduced sufficiently, a further dose should be given, usually being 25% of the original dose. The difficulty comes in knowing where to stop and it is easy for the inexperienced anaesthetist to end up with a patient too deeply or too lightly anaesthetized.

Mouth-opening

The loss of muscle tone under intravenous anaesthesia is extremely variable and, since virtually all dental procedures require the mouth to be open, various methods have been tried to overcome this problem. The first and oldest is to use some sort of gag which literally forces the teeth apart. They are without doubt effective but the high number of injuries resulting from careless handling makes their routine use undesirable. (They also suffer from the fact that they are unstable unless supported.) There is still a place for such gags in emergency situations and they are still advocated by some anaesthetists for use during inhalational anaesthetics.

The other method is to use a mouth prop of which there are many varieties. These can either be inserted prior to, or after induction. Prior insertion is uncomfortable but does ensure success and, providing the patient's jaw is supported until loss of consciousness, is the most satisfactory technique. Alternatively, it may be inserted when the patient is asleep by 'jerking' the patient's jaw firmly open.

Protecting the Airway

There is little doubt that patients protect their own airway better under light intravenous anaesthesia, than they do under inhalational anaesthesia. This should not induce complacency but rather a need for increased awareness since the less common incidents are the hardest to deal with. While the anaesthetist should ensure satisfactory cardiovascular and respiratory function, the dental surgeon can assist by minimizing the amount of blood, saliva or foreign material in the mouth. This is achieved by the use of careful techniques and by using high-volume low-pressure suction. It is also achieved by the use of mouth packs which can be gauze, sponge or foam. There is little doubt that the anatomically designed 'V' pack offers the best protection not just in terms of obtunding the mouth-to-pharynx passage but by supporting the tongue in a forward position (*see Fig. 3.12*).

The Use of Incremental Techniques

These have been mentioned in the text. They are not taught at an undergraduate level, but were pioneered by the late Drummond-Jackson. He suggested that the operator should administer the agent and that a trained assistant should observe the vital functions. The use of ultra-light anaesthesia and the so-called minimal increments is (at least statistically) relatively safe but it has on occasion been used with tragic results. Incremental techniques are useful and should be the subject of post-graduate training but their use is highly controversial in the realms of anaesthetic politics. Discussion of the details of such techniques is not apposite in this text, since it has no place in undergraduate teaching. The same is not true, however, of intravenous sedation and this is discussed in the following chapter.

CHAPTER 6

ORAL AND INTRAVENOUS SEDATION (INCLUDING PREMEDICATION)

While there can be little doubt that inhalational sedation is a useful and versatile technique, it does have distinct limitations. Not least of these is the need for a fair amount of patient co-operation and the not infrequent patient in whom the sedative effect is simply inadequate. Consequently a variety of oral and intravenous agents have been tried and tested with varying amounts of success.

The criteria for satisfactory sedation are those discussed in the previous chapter. Additionally, the agents themselves should be:

1. Easily administered.
2. Quickly effective.
3. Free of side-effects.
4. Of predictable duration and action.
5. Quickly metabolized or excreted.

Of this list the last four factors can be clearly related to the pharmacokinetics discussed in Chapter 2. In terms of intravenous agents the total volume of injected fluid clearly circulates in the blood until it is either redistributed, metabolized or excreted. Oral sedatives are less predictable in that they vary in relation to:

1. The degree of anxiety.
2. The amount and speed of absorption.
3. The rate of metabolism.

Thus the outcome of many oral sedative agents is less predictable than those given parenterally. Their advantages, however, are that they are usually well tolerated by most patients, they avoid the need for injections and their effect is usually longer lasting (though often milder) than their intravenous counterparts. Additionally, in younger children the oral premedicant can overcome the barriers of unreasoned irresponsibility which often exist in the first decade of life. To such children no amount of explaining will produce co-operative behaviour. This is not to say that premedication is essential, for confidence building can be developed through processes of repetition and reassurance, which given time may well produce satisfactory behaviour. In this realm it is still the belief of the authors that the formation of a treatment plan should proceed along the lines outlined in *Fig.* 1.1 (p. 2). Sedation or general anaesthesia should be reserved only for those patients for whom satisfactory treatment would not otherwise be possible. In the adult, sedation is usually only necessary because of fear and anxiety. In the words of Foreman (1974), 'Since its origins, dentistry has, more than any other of the health sciences, been intimately associated with anxiety, fear and pain'. It is the function of a sedative to allay fear and anxiety; if it also reduces pain, this is a supplementary beneficial effect. Satisfactory sedation should have the long-term aim of breaking the 'intimate association' described by Foreman, so allowing an improvement in the standard of dental health care. It is unfortunate that dentists have frequently misused sedatives to produce a semi-comatose patient on whom a large quantity of inadequate work can be quickly performed. In the anxious adult therefore the only justifiable use of sedation is to break down the barriers of fear and anxiety to reintroduce the patient to good dental care. In so doing the value of sedation is greatest for the earlier appointments and with skilful management its use can be decreased until it proves unnecessary.

Sedation in children is a somewhat different proposition. Irrational behaviour is not an uncommon feature in children under the age of ten, although behavioural responsibility is an extremely variable factor in a child's development. Certainly the influence of parents in their children's behaviour is unquestionable. Successful parenthood will commonly produce a confident self-assured child, who will react favourably even in new and potentially threatening situations. Anxious or disinterested parents on the other hand usually manage to instil a feeling of fear and mistrust which is, to say the least, difficult to counter.

Confident, self-assured and sympathetic handling is most likely to break this behaviour pattern. It is the dental surgeon who must assess the demands he can acceptably make on a child and, having given an instruction, it must be fulfilled in order to build confidence in the relationship. The situation is the same for the anaesthetist since there are basically only two ways of accomplishing treatment: by force or by agreement. It may be felt by some that sedation is an acceptable compromise between the two possibilities.

As the child nears the end of his first decade he becomes more rational and therefore more open to reason. There are still vivid exceptions to this general rule, but the behaviour patterns of the older child are somewhat different. Some of course are still fearful, but more often as a result of bad experiences in their younger years or as a result of hearing of such experiences from their friends or family. Such fear responds well to the anxiolytic drugs used in adults, though relatively higher dosages are often required.

Other children are plainly naughty in their behaviour. (Distinguishing this from fear is not always easy, but in general terms naughtiness is more commonly seen in front of parents and decreases on separation of the child from his parents.)

Strict discipline will usually allay naughtiness but sedation with a view to reducing activity rather than fear has a useful niche here.

ORAL SEDATION

Over the years various drugs have been tried as oral sedatives and some of them are examined below. The list is not exhaustive, but the major pharmacological groups of commonly used oral sedatives are included.

Diazepam

This is currently the most commonly and widely used sedative. It is a member of the benzodiazepine family, a large group of drugs with varying anxiolytic, sedative and hypnotic effects. It is usually available in tablets of 2 mg, 5 mg and 10 mg and is fairly reliably absorbed from the gut, its effect becoming apparent after 30 min. The actual required dosage is not easy to calculate since several factors influence its action. In particular, it does appear to bear a relationship to the age of a patient, much higher (relative) dosages being required in children and adolescents. The converse is true in the elderly. As a rough guide a dose between 0·1 and 0·25 mg/kg of body weight will produce adequate sedation and should be given 1 h before surgery and following a light snack. If there is any possibility that anaesthesia will be required, then no food or liquid should be taken preoperatively. (A small sip of water may be consumed for the purpose of swallowing the pills.)

Administration of a single dose of oral diazepam does give the operator the opportunity to form a baseline assessment on which further action may be based. Too high dosage will cause sleep, whilst inadequate dosage will result in an alert and still anxious patient. Potential side-effects include dizziness, increased pain awareness, ataxia and occasional respiratory depression. Prolonged postoperative drowsiness has also been reported.

Caution is necessary in administering diazepam to patients with obvious psychoses, neuromuscular disorders, respiratory disease and liver or kidney disease. Alcohol intake must be prohibited for a period of 24 h before and after administration. Patients should not drive or operate machinery for 24 h post-medication.

Oral diazepam has been found particularly useful in the treatment of spastic patients, coupling it with intravenous injection in severe cases. (Use of intravenous diazepam is considered later in this chapter.)

Temazepam and Lorazepam

Temazepam has been generally marketed as a hypnotic but it has been found very useful as a sedative. Like diazepam it is a member of the benzodiazepine family but it has the advantage of a relatively short half-life. In terms of its use as a hypnotic this makes any 'hangover' effect virtually non-existent. Used as a sedative it produces fairly rapid relaxation, its anxiolytic properties being very good. It is more expensive than diazepam and has no advantage, if intravenous supplements are anticipated. Where oral sedation is sufficient, however, its short half-life makes it a useful drug for use, particularly in adult patients, where the slowish recovery from diazepam can be a little disturbing. In general terms, the precautions and side-effects are the same as those mentioned above for diazepam. The usual dosage is 10–30 mg for the healthy adult, care being taken not to give too high a dose which will result in sleep.

Lorazepam is another hypnotic which has also been used for pre-operative sedation, though it does not appear to have gained wide acceptance. Its action is similar to diazepam and an intravenous injectable form is available. It is not particularly suitable for use in children but provides satisfactory sedation in adults with doses between 1 and 4 mg depending on the degree of anxiety. As with most benzodiazepines the therapeutic dosage normally decreases with age.

The Barbiturates

The use of barbiturates has been almost entirely supplanted by the benzodiazepines and there is now very little indication for their use in preoperative sedation. Occasionally, the use of pentobarbitone sodium is encountered but it can really only be justified in patients who are hypersensitive to benzodiazepines. Drug tolerance and dependence easily occur with all barbiturates. Additionally, their use in cases of respiratory, renal or hepatic disease should be avoided and the concomitant use of any other central nervous system depressants is contra-indicated. Under no circumstances should oral barbiturates be given to patients in pain as they may cause confusion and irritability.

Trimeprazine and Promethazine

Both these drugs are effective H1—histamine antagonists (anti-histamines of the phenothiazine group) and trimeprazine has been found particularly suitable for sedation in children. It is available in tablet or syrup form and has a reasonable anti-emetic action. It should be given in doses of about 2 mg/kg of body weight initially as higher doses may produce sleep. If the effect is inadequate at this level an increase of 50% of the initial dose should be given. Trimeprazine will often overcome the irrational fear found in younger children, which is often resistant to small doses of diazepam. This is therefore particularly useful for outpatient sedation, but in hospital where patients can be observed higher doses of diazepam are usually preferred. (In the hospital situation the phenothiazines may also be given in higher doses.) The side-effects of trimeprazine include persistent drowsiness, disturbing dreams (or other psychosomatic effects), nasal stuffiness and headaches. Occasional skin rashes and respiratory depression have been reported.

Promethazine hydrochloride has also been used in the sedation of children, but its use as a sole agent in sedation is less satisfactory than that of trimeprazine. Doses of 5 to 25 mg can be given orally from the age of 6 months to 10 years. Occasionally promethazine has reversed effects producing restlessness, irritability and hallucinations. Fortunately, this is extremely rare at the recommended doses.

The phenothiazines are a useful group of drugs which have a useful sedative action. This can be employed to great advantage in young children; in particular trimeprazine is extremely effective in calming an anxious child.

Triclofos

This is another useful sedative/hypnotic in a non-barbiturate group. It is derived from an old hypnotic known as chloral hydrate. Unlike the latter, however, it is virtually tasteless. It derives its effect as a result of hydrolysis within the body, when it breaks down into trichloroethanol. It is this metabolite which produces the hypnotic/sedative results. In addition, it is further metabolized and excreted relatively quickly, thus giving a relatively short half-life and infrequent 'hangovers'. It has little if any tendency to cause respiratory depression and is therefore useful in patients where it is mandatory to avoid this. For children over 1 year of age, a dose of 250 mg may be sufficient, but doses up to 500 mg may prove necessary in older children. Above the age of 6 years, this may be increased to 1 g in the severely anxious, but such high doses occasionally result in non-disturbable sleep.

Triclofos is potentiated in the presence of alcohol, barbiturates, CNS depressants and certain other sedatives and tranquillizers. It may also increase the potency of the coumarin type anti-coagulants and for this reason it should be avoided as a sedative in patients who are receiving these drugs.

Side-effects may include dizziness, headache and gastrointestinal upsets but the drug is relatively free of serious complications. It is contra-indicated in patients with severe renal, hepatic or cardiac impairment. Triclofos is no longer a commonly used drug, particularly in outpatients, but this is more due to the advent of the newer hypnosedatives, rather than to its lack of efficiency which is basically quite satisfactory.

The use of oral sedatives as premedicants is discussed in the section on premedication at the end of this chapter.

INTRAVENOUS SEDATION

It is the use of intravenous sedation which has developed most quickly over the past two decades in the treatment of nervous patients. This is particularly the case since intravenous diazepam was introduced in the mid 1960s, as it provided an extremely useful drug with a wide safety margin when used correctly. In the 10 years following its introduction the number of general anaesthetics administered within the NHS fell by around 25% in actual terms and by about 40% in terms of anaesthetics administered per treatment. This, of course, is part of a general trend and cannot be ascribed solely to the development of intravenous sedation though there can be little doubt that it has provided an acceptable alternative to general anaesthesia for a large number of patients and administrators.

Intravenous sedation was pioneered as far back as the mid 1940s by Professor Niels Jorgensen. The method he described (which became known as the Jorgensen technique) was to administer 10 mg pentobarbitone every 30 s through an intravenous cannula. When the patient becomes relaxed and at ease the dose given is noted and is termed the baseline dosage. The usual maximum in the healthy adult patient required to achieve the baseline is 100 mg and smaller doses are frequently successful. A further 10–20% of the baseline dosage is then injected followed by pethidine 25 mg and hyoscine 0·32 mg diluted to 5 ml. This is also given in proportion to the baseline dosage, i.e. if the baseline was achieved with 50 mg pentobarbitone, only 2·5 ml of the pethidine/hyoscine mixture is injected.

There is little doubt that the Jorgensen technique would have had a more universal acceptance, had it not been for three factors. First, the method is slow and requires a fair amount of experience in using it successfully. Secondly, a number of patients fall asleep, and while it is probably safe to operate on them the suppression of protective reflexes is unpredictable and so it must be avoided. Finally, the recovery time is exceedingly slow so the method is of dubious suitability as an outpatient procedure. Despite these factors there is little doubt that it was Jorgensen's work in this field which has led to the use of modern intravenous sedative techniques. It is particularly the search for a safely operator-administrable sedative which has been the focus of most research.

In this realm it is important to reconsider the minimal incremental technique first described by the late Drummond-Jackson in 1965. This employed the use of the ultra-short acting methylated oxybarbiturate—methohexitone given intravenously to a baseline level and then supported periodically by increments as small as possible to maintain 'sedation', or ultra-light anaesthesia. The hypothesis in this situation is that although the patient is asleep and psycho-somatically unaware, he does still have the full use of his protective reflexes. It was therefore claimed to be suitable for use by an operator and one or two trained assistants.

Those who have used methohexitone in the circumstances would have to agree that the effects described by Drummond-Jackson are largely true.

They do vary markedly, not just from patient to patient, but also within one attempt at the technique. Independent research teams have demonstrated this variability and, in particular, noted a fair incidence of hypoxia associated with loss of control of the airway.

It is necessary, therefore, to condemn the use of methohexitone by an operator/anaesthetist, but in our view it may still have a place in the presence of a trained anaesthetist, who can constantly and without restriction observe the state of his patient (*see* Chapter 4). The use of other agents in variations of the incremental technique has involved althesin, propanidid and ketamine but the results are variable and they appear to offer no fundamental advantages.

Consequently the introduction of the intravenous benzodiazepines in the mid 1960s marked a major break-through. Reliable sedation without loss of consciousness can be virtually guaranteed in normal (but anxious) patients, permitting good patient co-operation, allowing continuous verbal contact and producing marked anterograde amnesia, particularly in the first few minutes after the injection. The normal duration of sedation is around half an hour, though the recovery is so gentle that it is often possible to continue treatment for some time even after the effect has worn down. This is particularly the case if the procedure involves no pain and encroaching into this end period often proves a satisfactory way of helping the patient to sedation free treatment. If a longer period of sedation is required this can be achieved by giving the intravenous diazepam on top of a premedicating loading dose given 1 h preoperatively.

Method of Administration

Intravenous diazepam is an oily fluid with a marked tendency to produce thrombophlebitis. This can be minimized by injecting it into a large vein, usually in the ante-cubital fossa. Upon registering a satisfactory aspiration the diazepam is slowly injected at a rate of not more than 1 ml (5 mg)/min. During the period of the injection continuous conversation is kept between the patient and the operator. Slight slurring of the patient's speech is often the first sign of approaching therapeutic levels. Additionally, observation of the upper eyelid will show a degree of ptosis which bisects the pupil when satisfactory sedation is achieved (*Fig.* 6.1). The total dose varies from patient to patient quite considerably throughout a range of some 5–20 mg. Occasionally giggling or crying reactions occur for no apparent reason. These are probably due to the diazepam releasing the patient's emotions which then become exaggerated. It can usually be overcome by increasing the dose administered by another 25%.

The peak amnesic effect occurs about 1 min after injection and at this stage intra-oral local anaesthetics should be administered. The degree of relaxation may produce an increased reaction to painful stimuli so the patient should be warned to keep still and that he may experience pain. Topical anaesthetics can be useful in reducing untoward reactions.

Complications following intravenous diazepam are relatively rare. Occasional apnoea occurs though this is frequently a result of prior nervous hyperventilation and is more correctly termed respiratory depression. It is rare for such patients to develop cyanosis. A genuine apnoeic reaction may require the patient to be ventilated with oxygen which should always be instantly available.

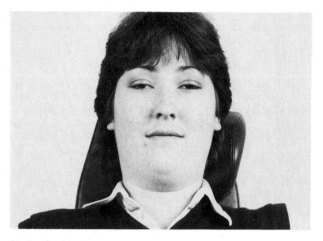

Fig. 6.1. Ptosis with diazepam. Together with slurring of speech this represents the ideal level of satisfactory sedation.

Recovery is relatively slow though most practitioners allow their patients to return home 1 h after administration. Patients must of course be able to walk freely and be accompanied straight home. A rebound effect some 6–8 h later is not uncommon. The reason for this is not clear but it is probably due to the release of an active metabolite, desmethyl diazepine. Thus intravenous diazepam is more suitable for afternoon usage when patients can be sent home to recover until the next day. During this period patients should not drink alcohol, take any medication other than simple analgesics or essential medicines, not drive, operate machinery or involve themselves in any hazardous activity. Many patients report feeling normal 2 h postoperatively and then realizing the following day that their recovery was still incomplete.

The use of intravenous diazepam has been found successful in the treatment of mentally retarded patients and particularly spastic children, whose desire to co-operate is often inhibited by their involuntary physical movements. In the older child and adolescent exceptionally high doses are often necessary to provide satisfactory sedation. On occasions the required dose is higher than is acceptable with the desired safety margin. A half-sedated child can be harder to treat than a non-sedated one and a decision needs to be made to proceed to higher and possibly therapeutic levels or whether it would be more prudent to abandon treatment from the outset. In practice high doses of diazepam could be given safely but it is more efficacious to proceed to a general anaesthetic on a subsequent occasion. The usually recommended maximum dose for outpatient procedure is 20 mg of the intravenous agent but most patients require less.

Several attempts were made in the mid 1970s to produce a 'modified incremental technique' using methohexitone and diazepam together, but although they enjoyed some popularity they have not been widely accepted. Principally, however, the search for an adjuvant to be used alongside diazepam has been for an analgesic which could be given intravenously. In this context various drugs have been tried, in particular pentazocine which is a fairly potent opiate-like analgesic. The drug may potentiate the effect of the diazepam and there is at least one case on record of this combination being fatal. Other adjuvants have included morphine, pethidine and levorphanol.

The use of these potent analgesics essentially borders on a technique known as neuroleptanalgesia. This produces sedation with marked analgesia. Modern drugs used in this technique include droperidol and fentanyl. The latter is short acting, increments being required every 30 min or so.

It has been used for outpatient procedures using the same instructions as would be given for intravenous valium. A dose of 50 µg (1 ml) is the usual baseline for a healthy adult and increments of half this are given as necessary. It produces a warm, comfortable feeling in the patient with marked analgesia, which produces little reaction to the stimulus of intra-oral injection. Verbal contact is maintained with the patient and dental procedures should not be attempted if sleep occurs. A degree of anterograde amnesia appears to result but this is difficult to assess due to the decreased awareness to painful stimuli, resulting from the direct analgesia produced by the fentanyl.

The method used involves placing the patient in the supine position. The initial respiratory rate is then observed and is usually fairly rapid. Four millilitres of fentanyl are drawn up in a syringe to be administered conventionally through a butterfly needle in the hand or through one of the veins of the antecubital fossa. An initial dose of 1 ml is administered and any tendency to lowering of the respiratory rate in the next 30 s is observed. Assuming this does not occur a further 1 ml is administered. The patient is asked how the drug has affected him and a continuous patter of chat is maintained. Increments of 0·5 ml are added until the patient's speech slows and a relaxed if somewhat tired looking appearance develops. Throughout all this the respiratory rate is monitored, eight inhalations per minute being the absolute minimum before treatment, other than the administration of local anaesthetic, can begin. The risk of severe respiratory depression and its high cost does not commend fentanyl as a suitable drug for use by the operator/administrator. In practice, despite this depression of the respiratory rate, apnoea has not proved problematical and the respiratory rates of previously anxious patients has remained on the high side. The diminished reaction to the painful stimulus of the local anaesthetic is clearly noticeable though it is still usual for some reaction to occur. The effect of the fentanyl averages some 30 min but unlike diazepam increments can be given with good effect. Being in aqueous solution it also has none of the tendencies to cause venous thrombosis and subsequent thrombophlebitis.

Since this has been the major disadvantage of intravenous diazepam, the search has been underway for some time for water soluble benzodiazepines. These have recently become available as have the lipid emulsion diazepams. These drugs have the advantage of a shorter half-life and therefore should be free of the rebound effects that are commonly reported with diazepam in propylene glycol. A further advantage is their usefulness as intramuscular injection and their decreased tendency to thrombophlebitis. The serum levels of diazepam following intramuscular injection are not significantly different from those established by oral administration. The aqueous benzodiazepines, however, have similar serum concentrations in intravenous or intramuscular form 1 h after administration, which is the usual time for giving preoperative medication (*see below*).

The performance of dentistry under sedation does require a degree of skill which only comes with practice. It is an essential part of all the methods of true sedation that verbal contact be maintained with the patient, although verbal replies are not always possible or desirable. Additionally, there is some evidence that covering the eyes of patients who are sedated prolongs and intensifies the sedative effect, but this removes another reliable sign which the operator can repeatedly observe. Probably the most dependable way of maintaining contact is to give occasional commands for the patient to follow, rather than asking vague questions, the answering of which is hard to assess.

In any type of procedure, conservative or surgical, it is essential to have good suction. The use of the dental V-pack (described earlier) is often possible and certainly every effort should be made to avoid contaminating the airway for while the aim of all sedation is to totally preserve vital reflexes there can be little doubt that they are frequently, if minimally, depressed. It is virtually certain that as time passes untrained anaesthetists (be they dentally or medically qualified) will become unacceptable and the trend towards sedation will presumably increase. Statistics already suggest that this trend is occurring but it is difficult to get accurate figures as to the number of sedatives being administered. One can foresee that in the next decade major advances into methods of sedation and the use of sedatives will occur, and while general anaesthesia is taught for the purpose of making the student aware of its capabilities, it will be in practising sedation that the real emphasis will be made.

PREMEDICATION

Premedication may be defined as the administration of drugs before an anaesthetic with a view to facilitating the operation and anaesthesia. Premedication is therefore a clinical concept and the drugs used fall into different pharmacological categories. The main features required of premedication include:

1. Producing a relaxed, calm patient.
2. Reducing salivary and bronchial secretions.
3. Reducing the response to painful stimuli.
4. Reducing the risk of vomiting.

Three basic types of drugs are available in producing a calm patient. These are the narcotics, the hypno-sedatives and the tranquillizers. It should be noted, however, that 'narcotic' is a pharmacological term while hypno-sedative and tranquillizer are clinical terms. The demarcation of these different groups is therefore not easy and some of the more popular drugs are mentioned below.

The Opiates (narcotics)

These naturally occurring substances are basically alkaloids of opium—an extract of the wild poppy seed. Similar powerful synthetic forms are available each with its own individual variations in properties. In general terms each drug will to a greater or lesser extent relieve pain, produce sedation and produce a combination of stimulatory and depressant actions in the central nervous system.

In all the categories extreme action of the drugs may be regarded as side-effects (e.g. depression of the cough and laryngeal reflexes) and great care should be taken in administering them. It is also important to be aware of the addictive nature of the opiates, which is both physical and psychological. There is some evidence that the risk of addiction is at its lowest when these drugs are administered intramuscularly. Premedication is seldom necessary for the dental outpatient, but when it is required, there is no place for the opiates. For inpatient procedures however, they are in common usage, particularly morphine, pethidine and papaveretum. The main criticism is that it is illogical to give powerful analgesics to patients with minimal or no pain. Despite this they are popular with patients and anaesthetists alike.

Morphine

In its basic form it occurs as a natural alkaloid but is commercially available as the hydrochloride or sulphate. It is a powerful depressant of the cough reflex, pain response and respiratory rate. It stimulates the vomiting reflex and the action of the pupillary muscles of the eye. However, the production of euphoric feelings still makes morphine a popular premedicant when used in conjunction with an anti-emetic. A dose of 5–20 mg may be given but the standard dose for a healthy adult is 10 mg.

Papaveretum

Papaveretum is less powerful in its effects than morphine and is also said to have fewer side-effects. It does certainly appear to produce less nausea but it is difficult to assess whether this is because relatively smaller doses are given (normally 10–20 mg for adults). The actual mixture of papaveretum has an equivalent morphine content of half its actual weight. As with morphine it is usually given in conjunction with an anti-emetic.

Pethidine

Pethidine is a less powerful analgesic than either morphine or papaveretum (morphine is about ten times more effective). It is, however, one of the synthetic narcotics and has fewer side-effects than either morphine or papaveretum. A dose between 25 mg and 100 mg is given but an adjunct, usually of the phenothiazine group is commonly administered to ensure adequate sedation.

All the narcotics rely on the liver and kidneys for their breakdown and excretion so should not be administered to patients with known hepatic or renal disease. Pethidine (and probably the natural opiates) should be avoided in patients who are taking monoamine oxidase inhibitors as indirect drug interactions can occur. The opiates should also be avoided in many of the diseases mentioned in Chapter 1.

The Hypno-sedatives

It is probably true to say that virtually every drug in this category has been tried at some time as a premedicant. The effects of individual drugs vary, but as in sedation itself the benzodiazepines, and in particular diazepam, enjoy prime position in terms of popular usage. The drug has been used orally and intramuscularly though the latter practice has become less popular. Diazepam remains a dependable oral sedative which has excellent soporific effects but given this way it produces minimal amnesia. Given intramuscularly its action is less consistent and if parenteral use is required, immediate preoperative intravenous injection is preferable. This is a particularly useful technique when anaesthesia with ketamine is contemplated, as it will usually eliminate the vestibular and visual disturbances which commonly occur postoperatively.

The use of phenothiazines (which are usually regarded as major tranquillizers) in premedication is becoming less common. They are useful anti-emetics and are sometimes used in the preparation of patients with fractured jaws who are going to have their jaws fixed in the closed position with either intra-oral or extra-oral fixation. It is more usual nowadays to give such drugs postoperatively and give anaesthetic drugs which are themselves anti-emetic. Some anaesthetists still prefer the 'grand slam', giving a narcotic analgesic, an antihistamine and an anti-sialogogue.

The Anti-sialogogues

An anti-sialogogue is a drug which suppresses secretions of the salivary glands. The most common way of achieving this is to prevent the secretomotor action of acetyl choline. Two pharmacologically similar drugs, atropine and hyoscine, are used virtually exclusively in this area. Both are naturally occurring alkaloids not totally dissimilar from cocaine in their chemical formula. Despite their similarities in structure and in reducing secretomotor activity they do have some fundamentally different affects on the central nervous system.

In particular, the standard dose for a healthy adult of 0·6 mg of atropine given intramuscularly will cause an initial bradycardia of short duration, followed by a more prolonged tachycardia. For some reason intravenous injection less commonly results in the initial bradycardia. The anti-sialogogue effect of atropine is said by some to be less than that of hyoscine, but research has shown the difference to be insignificant. It also has the advantage of being available as an oral preparation.

The cardiovascular effects of hyoscine are far less marked than those of atropine and if a slight tachycardia occurs it seldom reaches a rate where arrhythmias may result (which is occasionally the case with atropine). Hyoscine has the advantage over atropine of causing 'twilight sleep' when used in association with the narcotic analgesics. This results in a fairly profound sedation and is often followed by a reasonable degree of analgesia.

Administering Premedication

The actual content of the mixture of premedicants and their method of administration is the responsibility of the anaesthetist. However, for practical reasons it is sometimes necessary for the dentist to prescribe or administer the drugs. The basis on which drugs are given should be determined following an assessment of the nature of the anaesthetic, the operation and the individual patient.

Wherever possible, it is better to avoid premedicating an outpatient. On the few occasions where it becomes necessary an oral combination 1 h preoperatively with a *small* sip of water is probably the most satisfactory. Oral premedication is also useful in children and patients with bleeding diatheses in whom injections must be avoided.

In the inpatient, intramuscular injection is most suitable. By far the most common combination is papaveretum 20 mg and hyoscine 0·4 mg being the dose for a healthy average adult male. Higher doses are seldom necessary though it is necessary to scale down the dose in smaller people.

Used carefully, premedication is a useful technique on which to base sound anaesthesia both during and after the anaesthetic. Carelessly used, it produces side- and after-effects, which are undesirable and frequently unpleasant.

CHAPTER 7

ENDOTRACHEAL ANAESTHESIA

Since the introduction of muscle relaxants into clinical practice, intubation of the larynx has become one of the most frequently employed procedures in anaesthesia, because it affords control over the airway and pulmonary ventilation without the need for deep anaesthesia. Its advantages in oral surgery, allowing generous surgical access whilst giving the anaesthetist control of the airway, should be obvious. Anaesthetic techniques involving intubation of the larynx have many indications and some contra-indications, which together with techniques and complications will be discussed.

INDICATIONS

The indications for the use of tracheal intubation in oral surgery are:
1. Securing a clear airway.
2. Controlling ventilation.
3. Improving surgical access.

Securing and Protecting the Airway
With a cuffed endotracheal tube *in situ* in the larynx, aspiration into the lungs of foreign matter either liquid (e.g. blood, pus or vomit) or solid (e.g. fractured crown, prosthesis, amalgam etc.) is rendered less likely. The simultaneous use of an efficient throat pack placed in the pharynx prior to surgery is a 'belt and braces' approach to be recommended in any situation where foreign debris is to be expected in the pharynx, as the pack material employed (usually stout gauze or sponge foam) will provide a mechanical barrier to solid matter. It will also absorb any liquid lying in or entering the pharynx thus preventing pooling of liquid immediately above the vocal cords. Although the inflated cuff of the endotracheal tube might prevent such liquid material from gaining access to the lower respiratory tract during surgery, cuff deflation prior to extubation would allow entry into the trachea, especially if clearance, by suction, of the oropharynx had been either inadequate or omitted.

Two important points to be emphasized are that the stomach and its contents are a source of dangerous material to be aspirated, and that the presence of a cuffed endotracheal tube and a throat pack does not absolutely guarantee a protected airway, as liquid in particular can seep past the cuff into the trachea. The precautions routinely taken to allow gastric emptying in non-urgent cases prior to inducing endotracheal anaesthesia should always be enforced.

Improved Surgical Access

It should be obvious that during anaesthesia for dental surgery the operator and the anaesthetist are both working in the same anatomical area, i.e. they are sharing the airway. Endotracheal intubation allows surgical access to the oral cavity, enabling the anaesthetist to control an isolated airway. Nasal intubation allows the operator greater access and is therefore used routinely in oral surgery unless contra-indicated.

Control of Ventilation

The presence of an endotracheal tube allows the anaesthetist to control the patient's ventilation, particularly if a non-depolarizing relaxant has been administered in order to place the tube (*see below*). There are several advantages of controlled ventilation. Adequate muscle relaxation will allow a lighter plane of anaesthesia to be used which ensures a faster recovery. Carbon dioxide retention with its associated endogenous catecholamine secretion and cardiac arrhythmias will be minimized. It must also be noted that the presence of the endotracheal tube will effectively double the airway's resistance with a concomitant increase in the work of breathing. Although this may not be of great enough importance to influence the decision to ventilate an adult, it assumes greater importance when intubation is employed in children, as the material of the endotracheal tube itself will occupy a proportionately greater part of the cross-sectional area of the airway. Thus the bore of the airway will be smaller and present a greater resistance to air flow. In this situation intermittent positive pressure ventilation (IPPV) is necessary.

Control of ventilation is not essential in adults, particularly if the procedure is of short duration. Other disadvantages of controlling ventilation are that the patient's usual blood carbon dioxide level (Pa_{CO_2}) may be reduced, thus removing the stimulus for normal spontaneous respiration (*see* Chapter 2), thus delaying recovery. Furthermore, manual ventilation, i.e. by squeezing the anaesthetic reservoir bag, is likely to be irregular in both frequency and tidal volume, and few dental surgeries will run to the luxury of an automatic ventilator.

CONTRA-INDICATIONS TO ENDOTRACHEAL INTUBATION

Intubation of children under 10 years who are outpatients, i.e. they go home following surgery, should not be performed, as there is the risk of laryngeal and subglottic oedema following extubation causing airway obstruction. Although postoperative croup is uncommon, the prospect of risking total airway obstruction with the child having left the clinic to go home cannot be entertained.

Nasal intubation is contra-indicated in cases of grossly distorted nasal septum where excessive force may be required to pass the tube. In patients with disorders of blood coagulation, e.g. haemophiliacs, or patients taking anticoagulant drugs, the minor trauma of a normal nasal intubation can provoke bleeding which will be difficult to control.

Oral intubation may prove impossible in the presence of severe anatomical deformities of the mandible, temporomandibular joint or cervical spine. Examples in which attempts at oral intubation should be avoided include congenital deformities such as the Pierre Robin syndrome, and acquired disease of the temporomandibular joint or cervical vertebrae such as rheumatoid arthritis and ankylosing spondylitis. A skilled anaesthetist may well prove successful in intubation using spontaneous ventilation and the blind nasal technique. Muscle relaxants must *never* be used prior to intubation in patients with anatomical airway problems, as they will abolish the muscular activity necessary for spontaneous respiration. Should the patient then prove impossible to intubate, it may also be difficult to maintain ventilation with a face mask.

INTUBATION TECHNIQUES

There are two basic techniques employed in intubating the trachea:

1. Intubation by direct laryngoscopy, in which the larynx is visualized using a laryngoscope.
2. Blind nasal intubation in which no visualization of the larynx need take place.

Each technique employs a rather different anaesthetic approach and only the former will be discussed. Specialized techniques such as 'awake intubation' using topical local anaesthesia of the oropharynx and larynx will not be included. A short section on the clinical use of muscle relaxants is included at the end of the chapter.

Intubation by direct laryngoscopy is the commonest method of intubation and owes its widespread use to the rapid and profound muscle relaxation produced by the intravenous administration of a muscle relaxant drug. The equipment available (*Fig.* 7.1) for reliable and safe intubation should consist of:

1. An appropriate selection of endotracheal tubes in the sizes considered suitable for the proposed patient. A spare endotracheal tube at least one size smaller than the one anticipated should always be available, as the patient's larynx may prove too small to accept comfortably the tube initially selected. However, it is also important to pass as large a tube

as will safely fit the patient's larynx, as this will minimize the increase in airway resistance inevitably introduced by the tube itself. Since the resistance is inversely proportional to the square of the tube's cross-sectional area, this is of great significance.

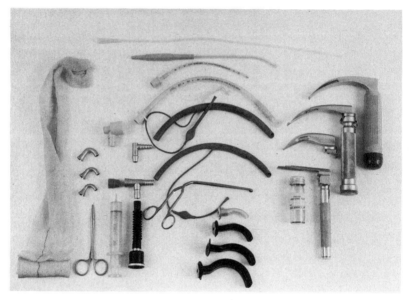

Fig. 7.1. The hardware required for routine intubation. Other equipment (e.g. an introducer) should also be available.

Various designs of endotracheal tubes are available constructed of either red rubber, polyvinyl chloride (PVC) or latex rubber. Although the selection of a particular tube type is not crucial, the most appropriate tube will often improve patient management. In brief, all tube materials are tested for tissue toxicity, but the modern PVC tubes are generally regarded as being the least irritant. Therefore, a PVC tube would be an appropriate choice for a prolonged surgical procedure. Similarly, all tubes can kink and obstruct the airway. However, latex rubber tubes, rendered relatively kink-proof by a spiral steel (or nylon) spring implanted in the wall of the tube so as to reinforce it, are indicated in situations in which head position renders kinking of the endotracheal tube more likely.

The design of the cuff of endotracheal tubes has been scrutinized carefully over the past decade. Since the aim of the cuff, when inflated, is to form a seal between the tube and the tracheal mucosa, pressure must be exerted by the cuff against the mucosa. In the case of the red rubber tubes the cuffs are of small volume and appose a small area against the tracheal mucosa. The pressure within these small cuffs is very high (up to 100 mmHg) and this pressure may produce ischaemia in the tracheal wall. The trend with more recently designed PVC endotracheal tubes is to use a cuff of large volume within which the pressure is low, and which presents a large surface area to the tracheal mucosa, thus reducing the likelihood of mucosal damage. The large area of contact also makes for a more efficient seal.

The endotracheal cuff is inflated using a syringe via a fine tube which passes from the cuff up the wall of the endotracheal tube to the mouth. This tube is glued to the wall of the endotracheal tube for most of its length. A short length of this fine bore tube at the mouth end hangs free in order to provide easy access for inflation. Along this free portion of the inflating tube (*Fig.* 7.2) is situated the pilot balloon. This small balloon communicates with the endotracheal cuff and the pressure which distends

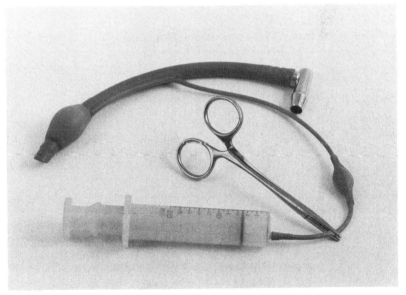

Fig. 7.2. A nasal endotracheal tube. The inflated cuff and pilot balloon can be seen.

the cuff also distends the pilot balloon. During cuff inflation, air is injected from the syringe into the cuff via the balloon, and the lungs are inflated via the endotracheal tube whilst listening carefully for an air leak around the cuff. Only sufficient air to just prevent a leak is injected into the cuff and the inflation tube is then clamped or plugged with its plastic bung. The pilot balloon, both by its distension, and the pressure within as detected by palpation, will give an indication of the pressure present in the endotracheal cuff. Too high a pilot balloon pressure can be caused by over enthusiastic inflation by the anaesthetist or selection of an inappropriate endotracheal tube size, i.e. if it is too small for the patient's trachea an excessive cuff inflation is required to stop air leaking. This only applies to adults, as in children it is mandatory to use a non-cuffed tube and allow a leak to occur. The pressure exerted by the cuff or too large a non-cuffed tube on the tracheal mucosa will encourage the development of laryngeal oedema which may compromise the airway following extubation.

2. An appropriate selection of laryngoscopes suitable in size and style for the proposed patients. Laryngoscopes are made in a variety of styles each with varied benefits. Essentially a laryngoscope is a modified battery-operated torch, the bulb of which provides illumination for a metal or plastic blade shaped in such a way as to enable the user to atraumatically displace the soft tissues of the floor of the mouth to give a suitable view of the larynx to be intubated. The laryngoscope blade must therefore provide enough room in the mouth and oropharynx not only for visualization of the cords, but also tube placement.

There are two styles of laryngoscope blade, curved and straight. The most commonly used blade in the UK is the curved MacIntosh blade designed by Sir Robert MacIntosh, Emeritus Professor of the Nuffield Department of Anaesthesia, Oxford. This blade is not only curved but also possesses a lateral step. The curve is designed to take the blade over the base of the tongue so that the tip slips anterior to the epiglottis into the vallecula. Gentle upward pressure in the vallecula then produces tension in the epiglottis, lifting it anteriorly to expose the rima glottidis and vocal cords. Introduced prior to the use of muscle relaxant drugs, this blade was designed to avoid contact with the sensitive mucous membrane on the dorsal aspect of the epiglottis thus making reflex laryngospasm less likely. The lateral step built into the blade pushes the tongue to the left of the oral cavity as the blade is passed down the right lingual sulcus (*Fig.* 7.3).

Several straight-bladed laryngoscopes exist, some with a small terminal curve of the blade, all of which were designed to lift up the epiglottis by direct contact with its dorsal surface (*Fig.* 7.1). This is particularly necessary in infants in whom the epiglottis is particularly floppy.

Regardless of the instrument preferred by the anaesthetist, it is most important to have a spare working laryngoscope always at hand. If the one instrument in use fails, another is immediately ready for use. This is particularly important during emergencies. Causes of laryngoscope failure include loose bulb, bulb failure, faulty connection between handle and blade, and of course, dead batteries. It should go without saying, therefore, that spare bulbs and batteries should be available, but most importantly that both laryngoscopes should be tested prior to anaesthetizing every patient.

3. Adequate suction apparatus must be available and tested prior to the

ENDOTRACHEAL ANAESTHESIA

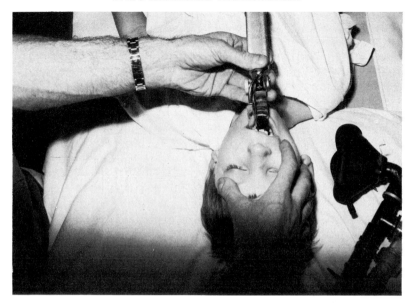

Fig. 7.3. Laryngoscopy prior to intubation. Having positioned the head initially, the right hand supports the upper lip and the little finger of the left hand the lower lip. The tongue is then displaced to the left by the blade.

administration of the anaesthetic, especially for intubation anaesthesia where the use of the muscle relaxant drugs deprive the patient of the muscle power necessary to protect the airway. Not only will secretions need to be removed to protect the airway, but their clearance may help in clearly visualizing the larynx. Large volumes of fluid, e.g. vomit, blood or regurgitated gastric contents, very occasionally present during laryngoscopy prior to intubation. The suction apparatus available in most anaesthetic induction rooms will not be able to remove such dangerous material quickly enough, particularly if solid matter is present, as the bore of the tubing and the flow rate through the apparatus is often inadequate. High-volume, low-pressure suction is essential for safe anaesthesia.

4. The chair or operating table upon which the patient is anaesthetized must be capable of quickly placing the patient completely flat or in a head-down position, if required. In instances where vomiting or regurgitation occurs head-down tilt with the patient in the lateral position will encourage drainage of the vomitus out of the mouth and away from the respiratory tract.

5. A large and small pair of Magill's forceps will be needed to pack the oropharynx following intubation (*Fig.* 7.4) and to remove the pack prior to extubation. It is also possible that a foreign body can be successfully removed from the pharynx using them. The forceps possess two 90° bends,

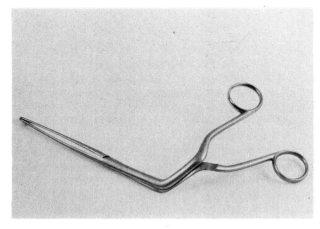

Fig. 7.4. Magill's forceps. They are curved through two different planes to give easy access to the pharynx in placing tubes and packs.

one which takes them into the oral cavity, and the second which directs the grasping arms of the forceps down into the pharynx. A laryngeal spray to spray the larynx and vocal cords with topical local anaesthetic is not an essential piece of equipment, though they are commonly available.

The required equipment in terms of oxygen, anaesthetic circuit, airways and masks has been discussed in Chapter 3 and the requirements do not differ during endotracheal anaesthesia.

Successful intubation of the patient's larynx under general anaesthesia requires the following:

1. The patient must be asleep. Although awake intubation is possible, the technique is beyond the scope of this book.

2. Sufficient relaxation of the patient's muscles must be obtained to allow the atraumatic adjustment of the anatomy of the upper airway, i.e. movement of the mandible and distortion of the soft tissues of the floor of the mouth, in order to visualize the larynx. Relaxation of the vocal cords will facilitate the passage of the tube between them. The manner in which one achieves these requirements varies from the use of a single drug or inhalational agent, to a combination of several.

In the past both intravenous and inhalational agents have been used to produce anaesthesia with sufficient muscle relaxation. Prior to the introduction of the muscle relaxant drugs, there were essentially two suitable agents capable of producing intubation conditions. Diethyl ether, the inhalation general anaesthetic, produces good muscle relaxation in the deeper planes of anaesthesia. However, in order to obtain the depth of anaesthesia required for intubation, the patient suffered a prolonged and sometimes stormy induction. Recovery was slow and often associated with unpleasant side-effects. Consequently, the technique is now rarely used. The intravenous induction agent thiopentone sodium has been used in high dosage to provide intubating conditions. The dosage required to depress the central nervous system sufficiently to obtain muscle relaxation also causes dangerous myocardial depression and its use in this manner has been abandoned.

Unfortunately inhalational or intravenous drugs used alone in high dosage in an attempt to produce intubating conditions always produce undesirable side-effects. Therefore, a combination of drugs is used, each drug being used within its appropriate dose range and chosen for its specific effect.

Most currently employed anaesthetic régimes aim to produce hypnosis, using either a modern inhalation agent or a modern intravenous induction agent, and then muscle relaxation using one of the currently available neuromuscular blocking drugs.

Intubation in children is, however, often undertaken using an inhalation technique as the necessary muscle relaxation is achieved more easily than in adults.

Visualization of the Vocal Cords

Since light travels in straight lines, it follows that in order to visualize the larynx and vocal cords using a conventional laryngoscope it will be necessary to manipulate the anatomical position of the tissues so that the axis of the oral cavity, the pharynx and the larynx lie in the same straight line. From the upper incisor teeth the longitudinal axis of the oral cavity lies at almost 90° to the axis of the pharynx and larynx (*Fig.* 7.5).

To create the required straight line the pharyngeal axis is brought into the line of the larynx by flexing the cervical vertebrae. The axis of the oral cavity is adjusted to align it with that of the larynx/pharynx by extending the head on the atlas vertebrae. The blade of the laryngoscope helps in this manoeuvre by gently but firmly distorting the floor of the mouth, the tongue being displaced to the left and the soft tissues being displaced anteriorly.

Using a MacIntosh laryngoscope with a curved blade, the laryngoscope should be held in the left hand from the start of the laryngoscopy. Transferring the instrument from one hand to the other in the patient's mouth is to be discouraged, as it can result in unnecessary trauma. The right hand controls the head and is used to open the mouth while the left hand carefully inserts the blade of the laryngoscope between the teeth and down the right lingual sulcus displacing the tongue to the left. Lubrication of the blade is sometimes a help, particularly if the patient has a dry mouth. Continuous observation of the anatomical landmarks during the introduction of the laryngoscope helps both in preventing trauma to the tissues, and in achieving a clear view of the larynx and vocal cords prior to introducing the endotracheal tube. At the back of the oral cavity the

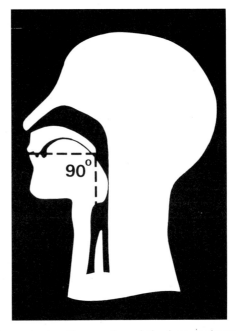

Fig. 7.5. Diagram to show the normal angulation between the mouth and the trachea.

uvula, hanging down from the soft palate, will indicate the midline and as the tip of the laryngoscope blade slips over the base of the tongue the tip of the epiglottis should be visualized. The curve of the blade will then take the blade to the junction between the epiglottis and the base of the tongue where gentle pressure from the blade upwards along the line of the handle will cause the epiglottis to be pulled anteriorly to expose the laryngeal inlet and the vocal cords.

Prior to introducing the endotracheal tube the vocal cords and laryngeal inlet can be sprayed with topical anaesthetic solution using an atomizer spray. Lignocaine 4% topical anaesthetic solution in a dose of 2 mg/kg is appropriate and this dose should not be exceeded, as the absorption of the drug across the mucous membrane is sufficiently rapid to produce toxic blood levels. Topical anaesthesia of the vocal cords and larynx is contra-indicated in patients in whom the oropharynx will contain potential foreign matter during recovery (e.g. blood, teeth, fragments, amalgam etc.), as the loss of sensation induced by the topical anaesthesia, if it persists into the recovery period, will make aspiration of a foreign body more likely.

The endotracheal tube itself should be lubricated with a clear non-irritant water-soluble jelly applied thinly to the portion of the tube which will lie at and below the vocal cords. This will reduce the friction between the laryngeal mucosa and the tube during its passage through the larynx and the tube will be better tolerated. The inbuilt curve of most endotracheal tubes allows the tube to lie comfortably in the cavity of the larynx, oropharynx and mouth or nose. This curve is also important in allowing the tube to be passed in from the side of the mouth thus giving an unobstructed view of the larynx in the midline. Occasionally a particularly soft tube will have insufficient curve in order to fit the patient's anatomy. In this situation a blunt-tipped stylette, usually made of a malleable material such as copper, is passed down the tube, and bent into the correct shape. The stylette must be lubricated to allow easy removal after tube placement and its tip must never extend beyond the end of the endotracheal tube. The stylette must never be used to push the tube forcibly past the cords into the larynx.

Causes of a difficult laryngoscopy and intubation may lie with the anaesthetist and his technique, or with the patient. Experience and practice will lower the frequency of failure due to poor technique, and careful patient assessment will select those patients in whom problems can be anticipated.

There are essentially four major failures of technique which can cause intubation problems:

1. The patient is inadequately anaesthetized or paralysed. This will give rise to difficulties in positioning the patient's head and neck for intubation, and will make laryngoscopy difficult due to the inability of the anaesthetist to displace the soft tissues with the laryngoscope. Force should never be used to overcome this problem. The anaesthetist should temporarily abort the attempted intubation, clear and maintain the airway, using artificial ventilation to maintain oxygenation, and ensure adequate anaesthesia and muscle relaxation prior to a further attempt at intubation.

2. The patient has been inadequately positioned for the attempted intubation. Care must be taken to correctly position the head, which should be extended on the upper cervical vertebrae while the neck is flexed. This is traditionally described as 'sniffing the morning air' (*Fig. 7.6*).

3. The anaesthetist has failed to observe the appropriate anatomical landmarks during laryngoscopy and the passage of the tube between the vocal cords. Practice and training improve this aspect of technique.

4. The choice of an inappropriately sized endotracheal tube, particularly in children, will render intubation difficult. Selection of too large a tube is usually the cause. Similarly, adjustment to the curvature of the tube may be needed in order to direct the tip of the tube into the larynx.

Patients may be difficult to intubate due either to:
    1. The size and shape of their airway anatomy.
    2. To the lack of mobility of the tissues.

1. Size and shape problems can be either congenital or acquired.

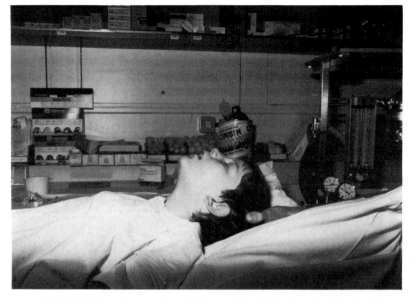

Fig. 7.6. 'Sniffing the morning air'. The neck is slightly flexed and the head extended.

Congenital causes include the classic example of the Pierre Robin syndrome with micrognathia, but any abnormality of the anatomy of the oropharynx or facial structure asssociated with the airway can cause problems, e.g. macroglossia.

An example of an acquired anatomical problem would be acromegaly in which not only the growth of the mandible presents a problem, but also the tissues of the larynx become distorted under the influence of excess growth hormone. Similarly, tumours of the tongue and larynx might be expected to pose problems as occasionally does tonsillar hypertrophy in children.

2. Mobility of the temporomandibular joint, the atlanto-occipital joint and the cervical spine is important in facilitating intubation. Acquired disease usually accounts for problems in reduced joint mobility, and specific enquiry must be made during patient evaluation, for rheumatoid arthritis, ankylosing spondylitis and temporomandibular joint abnormalities. Trismus caused by intra-oral pathology will be another source of difficulty. A further problem of tissue mobility which should be obvious on inspection of the patient will be severe skin scarring due to burns.

The most effective way of dealing with problems which cause difficult intubation is to anticipate them. This can only be done by rigorously examining each patient prior to inducing anaesthesia. Every prospective intubation patient should be asked about bone and joint disease, and carefully evaluated for mobility of jaw, head and neck. Size and shape of the teeth, maxilla and jaw should be noted with a view to excluding difficulties during intubation. Eternal vigilance is required.

Removal of the endotracheal tube at the end of an anaesthetic requires as much care as placing it at the beginning. Under direct laryngoscopy the oral or pharyngeal pack must be removed and the pharynx and laryngeal inlet cleared of debris by efficient suction. Adequate clearance of secretions and solid material prior to extubation will not only reduce the incidence of obstruction due to a foreign body in the airway, but will remove material capable of stimulating the laryngeal reflexes with subsequent laryngospasm. Should it be necessary, secretions must be aspirated from within the tube and trachea using a sterile suction catheter.

The moment at which to extubate requires careful judgement. If the patient has been breathing spontaneously using an inhalational agent it is possible to extubate the patient either when he is still deeply anaesthetized or when he is almost awake. The advantages of deep anaesthesia for extubation are that the patient recalls nothing of the extubation, the laryngeal reflexes are suppressed (making laryngospasm less likely) and the patient is also less likely to cough and strain. The disadvantages are that the patient will be totally unable to maintain and protect his own airway, respiration will be depressed and therefore a prolonged period of supervision during recovery will be required.

The advantages of extubation when the patient is almost awake are that recovery of the protective airway reflexes is almost complete, respiratory depression will be minimal, and the prolonged recovery period will be unnecessary. The risk of laryngospasm following removal of the tube in a lightly anaesthetized patient can be minimized by careful pharyngeal toilet, and by ensuring that the patient is as light as possible. An oropharyngeal airway should be placed in the mouth prior to extubation since it may be impossible to insert the airway if it is required when the patient's jaws are clamped firmly shut following the noxious stimulus of extubation.

Following muscle relaxant anaesthesia the major requirement is that the patient be fully reversed from the effects of the relaxant and has recovered sufficient muscle power for adequate ventilation—sufficient to produce a good cough as this is essential to protect the airway.

Prior to extubation, especially if nitrous oxide has been used, 100% oxygen should be given for 2–3 min. This pre-oxygenation will avoid diffusion hypoxia (*see* Chapter 2) as the relatively insoluble nitrous oxide pours out of the blood stream into the lungs, and will also provide a margin of safety should difficulty be experienced in maintaining the airway. Immediately before the tube is removed from the trachea the cuff, if present, should be deflated and the patient's lungs inflated with a generous breath by manually squeezing the reservoir bag of the anaesthetic machine. At full lung inflation the tube is removed and any secretions present in the laryngeal inlet will be expelled from the airway by the rush of oxygen out of the patient's lung. This manoeuvre can best be described as an artificial cough.

COMPLICATIONS OF ENDOTRACHEAL INTUBATION

Complications can arise during three stages of endotracheal anaesthesia. These are:
1. Those arising during the attempted intubation.
2. Those arising whilst the endotracheal tube is *in situ*.
3. Those arising following the removal of the endotracheal tube.

Attempted Intubation

Complications arising during the attempt at intubation are largely due to trauma. The nature of the complication varies with the technique of intubation used, be it nasal or oral.

During nasal intubation the nasal mucous membranes are always traumatized in some degree. Local bleeding of minor significance is the usual result, but local disease in the mucosa, such as infection, or a systemic bleeding tendency will render the bleeding more serious. Those conditions are therefore relative contra-indications to nasal intubation. Similarly trauma to the nasal septum sometimes occurs, particularly if previous injury to the nose has caused deviation of the nasal septum.

Occasionally during its passage backwards along the nasal cavity the tip of the endotracheal tube will fail to negotiate the curve of the nasopharynx. Forcing the tube at this point will result in the tube penetrating the mucosa and creating a false passage beneath the mucosa in the posterior wall of the pharynx. As long as this condition is recognized (usually by direct laryngoscopy and observation of the posterior pharyngeal wall) there are usually no major sequelae other than local bleeding. The endotracheal tube can usually be passed through the other nostril if it persists in following the submucous route in the nostril of first choice. Prior warming of the tube in hot water will soften the PVC tubes and make submucosal passage less likely.

Minor trauma to the adenoids in the nasopharynx is common during nasal intubation in children up to puberty, after which age the adenoids tend to atrophy.

Blind nasal intubation by its very nature entails attempted passage of the tube through the vocal cords into the larynx without the benefit of laryngoscopy. This carries the theoretical risk of an increased incidence of vocal cord trauma, although there is no concrete evidence to suggest that this is significant.

ENDOTRACHEAL ANAESTHESIA

During laryngoscopy the use of the laryngoscope or other metal instruments (e.g. the Magill's forceps commonly used to place the pharyngeal pack) carries with it the risk of trauma to the teeth and the oropharyngeal mucosa. Dental trauma usually takes the form of chipped enamel or very occasionally a fractured crown or a whole tooth being knocked out. Such incidents will be more common in patients with porcelain crowned incisors, patients with chronic periodontal disease and during difficult intubations. Occasionally, the Magill's forceps will cause mucosal tears, particularly on or around the uvula as this gets in the way when the nasal tube is being manipulated with the Magill's forceps. Uneventful healing is virtually always the rule.

In Situ Complications

Complications arising whilst the tube is *in situ* occur either because the tube is in contact with the respiratory mucosa, or because the airway is compromised.

Postoperative sore throat is the commonest complication arising from the contact of the endotracheal tube with the larynx. Trauma to the cords will also contribute to this soreness. The factors which aggravate the effects of the tube upon the respiratory mucosa include the material from which the tube is constructed, the nature and degree of the inflation of the tube cuff, lubrication of the tube prior to insertion, and to a lesser degree, whether the patient breathes spontaneously or is artificially ventilated. A dry mucosa following an anti-sialogogue premedication will also contribute to a sore throat. The re-use of the red rubber tubes may also be a factor as there is the possible risk of contaminating the respiratory tract with irritant agents used in the cleaning and sterilizing of the tubes.

The introduction of the modern large-volume, low-pressure floppy cuffs on the PVC endotracheal tubes might at first sight appear to lessen the incidence of sore throat by causing less pressure on the laryngeal mucosa when *in situ*. However, the cuff material of these tubes tends to gather in pleats when the cuff is deflated, and thus passage through the cords is not as atraumatic as with the old fashioned rubber cuffs.

It has been argued that spontaneous respiration through an endotracheal tube causes less movement of the tube against the mucosa than does the pressure wave caused by intermittent positive pressure ventilation. There is no conclusive evidence that this leads to fewer sore throats and it is probable that skilful placement of a well lubricated endotracheal tube of the correct size in a well relaxed patient will do as much as anything to avoid postoperative sore throat. Rare sequelae of intubation include vocal cord granulomata.

Complications arising from airway obstruction whilst the tube is *in situ* can be life threatening. Kinking of the tube, over-inflation of the cuff with resultant herniation into the lumen and apposition of the end of the tube against the tracheal wall are all possible mechanisms causing either partial or complete obstruction. For this reason the airway pressure should always be measured during artificial ventilation with a ventilator. Similarly, the feel of the bag must always be noted during manual ventilation. Disconnection of the tube from the anaesthetic circuit while hidden beneath surgical drapes will also be detected by such monitoring. Prolonged disconnection in a spontaneously breathing patient will result in the patient waking up. In a patient paralysed by muscle relaxants the patient will suffer either hypoxic brain damage or will die, depending upon the length of the apnoea.

A further problem which will give rise to an increase in airway pressure is inadvertent intubation of one of the main bronchi, resulting in ventilation of only one lung. Although one lung anaesthesia is possible for specific thoracic operations, it is dangerous and unnecessary during oral surgery. Careful attention to the length of endotracheal tube and observation of the expansion of the chest wall during inflation of the lungs to ensure inflation of both lungs will help to detect this mistake and avoid a hypoxic anaesthetic. Listening to both sides of the chest for breath sounds with a stethoscope is mandatory following intubation in children, as the shorter distance from the trachea to the main bronchi results in an increased risk of inadvertent bronchial intubation.

The complications induced by long-term intubation will not be discussed but the most severe are laryngeal stenosis and other problems related to local pressure necrosis of the tracheal mucosa.

Removal of Endotracheal Tube

Complications following the removal of the endotracheal tube invariably concern the airway function. Airway obstruction is the commonest problem following extubation and may be due to laryngeal oedema, laryngospasm, accumulation of secretions or failure of the patient to maintain his own airway. Oedema of the larynx is more likely to be a problem in children where the relative area of the lumen of the larynx is small. Any encroachment on this lumen by oedema of the mucosa will critically increase the resistance to airflow. Upper respiratory tract infections in children increase the likelihood of laryngeal oedema as the mucosa is already inflamed prior to intubation.

MUSCLE RELAXANTS IN CLINICAL USE

There are two types of muscle relaxant available, (1) Depolarizing relaxants which cause depolarization of the motor end plate prior to producing relaxation and (2) non-depolarizing relaxants which do not depolarize the motor end plate prior to producing relaxation.

Depolarizing Muscle Relaxants

During normal muscular activity efferent impulses from the central nervous system travel down the motor fibres of the peripheral nerves as waves of depolarization. At the point at which the nerve fibres meet the muscle fibres is a specialized area of contact called the neuromuscular junction (*Fig.* 7.7). On reaching the neuromuscular junction the depolarization causes the release of the chemical transmitter acetyl choline

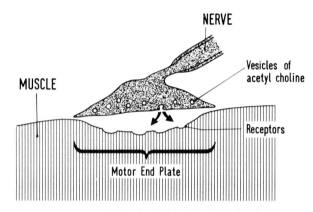

Fig. 7.7. The neuromuscular junction. The action of the depolarizing and non-depolarizing muscle relaxants on this structure is described in the text.

from the vesicles in which it is stored. The amount of acetyl choline released is determined by the number of pulses travelling down the nerve. The acetyl choline diffuses across the gap between the nerve ending and the muscle cell to an area called the motor end plate. The gap is very small (of the order of 1 μm) but the diffusion takes a finite time. On reaching the motor end plate the acetyl choline reacts with receptors to cause depolarization of the muscle fibres with subsequent contraction. Closely associated with the motor end plate receptors is the enzyme, acetyl choline esterase, which quickly removes the acetyl choline by breakdown into choline and acetic acid. This ensures that each muscular action is discrete and that the muscle contraction persists only as long as nerve impulses cause further release of acetyl choline.

The whole process is described by the term neuromuscular transmission and is fundamental to all voluntary muscle activity, the most important of which is breathing.

The only depolarizing relaxant available at present is suxamethonium. Chemically its structure is that of two molecules of acetyl choline joined together (*Fig.* 7.8). It is available in solution as the chloride salt in ampoules containing 100 mg in 2 ml and remains stable in solution if kept

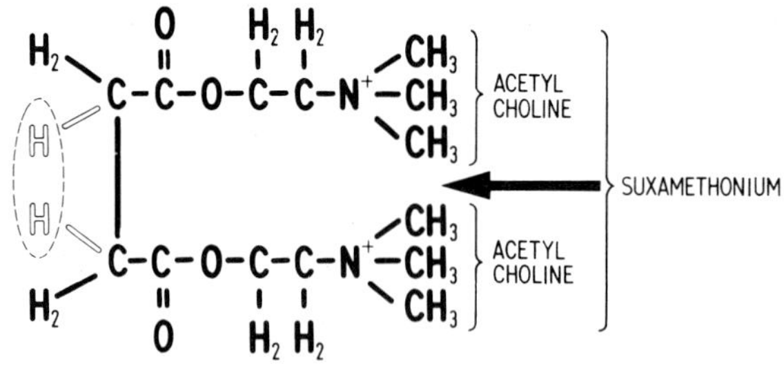

Fig. 7.8. The molecule of suxamethonium. The nature of its action is more clearly understood when its structural relationship to acetyl choline is considered.

refrigerated. High temperature and alkaline solution causes hydrolysis with loss of potency.

On intravenous injection in a dose of 1 mg/kg it causes widespread muscle fasciculation by depolarizing the motor end plates, i.e. its action is initially identical to acetyl choline. However, following depolarization the motor end plates are refractory and do not respond to acetyl choline released by the nerve endings. The onset of paralysis is rapid, profound muscle relaxation occurring within 1 min of injection and lasting from 3 to 5 min. Thus the main use of the drug is to quickly produce excellent intubating conditions. Recovery is rapid, as an enzyme in the plasma, pseudo-choline esterase, rapidly hydrolyses the drug removing one molecule of choline to produce succinyl monocholine and finally both molecules of choline to leave succinic acid. Genetically determined enzyme abnormalities render some patients incapable of hydrolysing the drug in the normal way and the length of action will be greatly prolonged. In this situation the patient will need to be kept asleep and artificially ventilated until muscle power returns. A family history of previous anaesthetic problems should be sought in the preoperative assessment though, fortunately, these cases are uncommon.

Side-effects of suxamethonium are generally related to its structural similarity to acetyl choline. The fasciculations produced by the drug give rise to muscle pains in the 24–48 h following the anaesthetic. These are worse in fit, muscular people. During the fasciculations the permeability of the muscle cell membranes is increased and potassium ions leak from the intracellular fluid out into the extracellular fluid. This movement of ions is accompanied, in the normal individual, by a rise in serum potassium of about 0·5 mmol/l which is insignificant. However, patients with a previously raised serum potassium and patients with severe burn, crush or denervation injuries are at risk of lethal rises in serum potassium, as the potassium influences myocardial contraction and the heart stops beating in asystole. In patients with muscular disease such as dystrophia myotonica the drug may paradoxically produce muscle spasm rather than relaxation. The above conditions should be considered contra-indications to the use of suxamethonium. Bradycardia is an occasional feature seen particularly when repeated doses of the drug are used to prolong relaxation. Heart rates below 60 beats per minute should be treated with intravenous atropine (0·6 mg). Rarely, suxamethonium provides the trigger for the condition known as malignant hyperpyrexia, in which the patient develops high temperature, tachycardia and becomes acidotic. Although rare the condition is genetically determined and a family history should be sought.

Non-depolarizing Muscle Relaxants

This group of relaxants act by successfully competing for the receptor sites on the motor end plate, thereby blocking the action of acetyl choline. They do not, however, depolarize the end plate (unlike suxamethonium) hence the adjective 'non-depolarizing'. In contrast to suxamethonium the typical features of the non-depolarizing muscle relaxants are that they:

1. Do not cause fasciculation.
2. Have a rather slower onset of action.
3. Produce a less profound relaxation.
4. Give a longer duration of muscle relaxation.

They are used for procedures expected to last 30 min or more. Endotracheal intubation and artificial ventilation usually with nitrous oxide and oxygen must be used as the muscles of respiration are always affected. Anaesthesia is supplemented by either low concentrations of a potent inhalational agent such as halothane or enflurane, or a potent intravenous narcotic such as fentanyl.

d-Tubocurarine is the oldest available non-depolarizing muscle relaxant first used in anaesthesia by Griffiths (1944). It is one of the naturally occurring alkaloids used by the South American Indians in their arrow poison (curare). Administered intravenously in a dose of about 0·5 mg/kg it produces good muscle relaxation in 3–4 min. The drug must not be administered as a bolus, but given over 30–45 s, as rapid injection can lead to sharp falls in the blood pressure due to histamine release and an autonomic ganglionic blockade. When used as the sole muscle relaxant the patient can be intubated after $2\frac{1}{2}$–3 min but artificial ventilation with a face mask and reservoir bag via the anaesthetic circuit will be required until intubation is achieved.

During surgical procedures further increments of curare of about 0·1–0·2 mg/kg can be given to maintain muscle relaxation, the need for which can be judged by the use of a nerve stimulator, or by observing muscle tone. Recurrence of spontaneous respiration is unlikely to be a useful sign as the patient is usually ventilated to a subnormal $Paco_2$ and the respiratory centre is also depressed by supplemental anaesthetic drugs. The inhalational agents halothane and enflurane interact with the muscle relaxant action of curare and the other non-depolarizing muscle relaxants to augment the neuromuscular blockade. Enflurane is more potent in this respect. Reversal of the curare neuromuscular blockade at the end of the surgery is easily achieved, particularly if only one dose of curare was given, and 25 or more minutes have elapsed since it was given.

Pancuronium is a synthetic steroid with potent non-depolarizing muscular blocking action which was introduced in 1967 and is now the most commonly used drug of its type in hospital practice. Administered intravenously in a dose of about 0·1 mg/kg its onset of action is marginally faster than curare, and patients may be intubated after $1\frac{1}{2}$–2 min. Its duration of action is rather longer than that of curare, a single dose lasting up to 45 min. Pancuronium does not produce the falls in blood pressure seen with curare, but it may be associated with a tachycardia as it blocks the vagus nerve in high dosage. Reversal of its action was considered a problem when it was first introduced but recognition of its potency and length of action have rendered reversal less of a problem. The drug is only suitable for hospital use.

Alcuronium is a semi-synthetic muscle relaxant which has been available since 1961. It is given in doses of the order of 0·2 mg/kg and its duration of action (up to 30 min) is marginally shorter than that of curare. It does possess some ganglion blocking properties, but the falls in blood pressure seen are less than with curare. Reversal of its action is hardly ever a problem.

Other non-depolarizing relaxants available but less commonly used include gallamine introduced in 1948 and other agents introduced in the past 5–10 years such as dacuronium, fazadinium and atracurium. The current quest by the pharmaceutical industry is for a non-accumulative non-depolarizing muscle relaxant with a duration of action of between 5 and 10 min and which has no cardiovascular side-effects. None of the agents so far produced has fulfilled these requirements.

Reversal of the (curare) neuromuscular blockade at the end of surgery is achieved using intravenous neostigmine, a cholinesterase inhibitor. Neostigmine prevents the breakdown, by acetylcholinesterase, of the acetyl choline released at the neuromuscular junction. This allows the acetyl choline to persist long enough to compete with the curare for the receptors of the motor end plate. Reversal of the blockade is made easier by the passage of time since the last dose of curare administered. Providing the time elapsed is longer than 20 min complete reversal is usually possible, particularly if only one dose of the agent has been given. Cases in which repeated doses of relaxant drugs have been given, i.e. the surgery has been prolonged, will require more time from the last dose of relaxant for full reversal to occur.

The dose of neostigmine employed is in the range of 40–60 µg/kg (0·04–0·06 mg/kg) and must be given with atropine in a dose of 20–30 µg/kg in order to avoid the muscarinic effects of the choline esterase inhibition. These effects may be both unpleasant, e.g. salivation, sweating and gastric intestinal colic, and dangerous, e.g. bradycardia.

The introduction of muscle relaxant drugs transformed anaesthetic practice by enabling intubation to be accomplished rapidly and easily. This widespread use of intubation has facilitated prolonged procedures and with the introduction of the short acting potent narcotic analgesics has reduced the requirement for high dosage inhalation anaesthesia to achieve muscle relaxation.

CHAPTER 8

COMPLICATIONS AND EMERGENCIES

The vast numbers of general anaesthetics (or sedatives) which are safely administered every day can easily lull one into a false sense of security. There are no short-cuts in anaesthesia. Sound technique must be based on adequate training both in the theoretical and practical aspects of the subject. In the vast majority of reported accidents the problems have arisen from a range of self-inflicted irresponsibilities, ranging from carelessness to total incompetence. It is not the basic methods that are responsible nor the drugs administered, but those who administer them who are usually at fault.

Consequently, it seems appropriate to re-emphasize here some of the lessons of Chapter 1. Preoperative assessment is an essential part of anaesthesia and care must be taken whenever any aspect of the patient's history suggests a problem. It is easy in this day and age for a medical opinion to be sought and short-cuts should never be taken as the consequences of any mistake may be so serious.

Even allowing for a reasonable standard of preoperative assessment there are cases where errors occur. For instance there is at least one death on record subsequent to a steroid crisis where the patient had been applying β-methasone cream to her skin too frequently. One can understand the practitioner's failure to elicit this fact preoperatively, but it cannot be denied that it probably cost the patient her life. Whilst such an example may be a rare and extreme case it nonetheless illustrates the fact that the method and drugs administered are only as reliable as those who administer them.

The range of complications is infinite, relating to either the dentistry or to the anaesthesia. They can extend from the smallest problem to the full-blown emergency, but in all cases one should aim primarily to avoid and secondarily to solve. Ignoring a problem is the quickest way to risk provoking an emergency, so if problems do develop, all dental surgery should be interrupted and the anaesthetist given full control.

Many of the factors in avoiding problems have already been mentioned in other chapters. Besides preoperative assessment the most important factor is the teamwork between the operator and the anaesthetist (or assistant in the case of sedative procedure). If both practitioners understand what the other is trying to achieve, and more particularly the relative importance of each others' efforts a harmonious and safe procedure will result.

It is assumed that in a hospital, all possible emergency facilities are available. In a dental surgery, however, there is a limit to the facilities

COMPLICATIONS AND EMERGENCIES

which can be provided and complicated resuscitation facilities are seldom seen. Indeed, without wide experience in their use items such as defibrillators and electrocardiograms are more likely to confuse the situation, rather than solve it. A list of suitable emergency drugs and equipment is listed below.

Adrenaline	Endotracheal tube + introducer
Aminophylline	Gag (for opening mouth)
Atropine	Intravenous cannulae
Calcium gluconate	Laryngoscope
Chlorpheniramine	Nasal airways
Dextrose drip	Oral airways
Diazepam	Reserve oxygen supply (*Fig.* 8.1)
Frusemide	Reserve suction supply
Hydrocortisone	Self-inflating resuscitator bag
Sodium bicarbonate	Tracheotome

All the drugs listed above have to be given by injection so appropriate syringes and needles should be in stock at all times.

The scouts' motto 'Be Prepared' is extremely relevant to dental anaesthesia. Because of the competition for the patient's airway, dentistry under general anaesthesia can be an extremely dangerous and risky procedure, and yet in practice it has had a relatively good safety record. 'Being prepared' is, however, only the beginning and one should seldom, if ever, have to resort to the use of emergency drugs. 'Being aware', is probably more appropriate to dental anaesthesia, and in particular the anaesthetist should:

1. Be aware of the patient's breathing pattern. Any obstruction should not be tolerated and air breathing quickly corrected.
2. Be aware of the patient's pulse. The temporal pulse, palpable in the pre-auricular region, is ideal. It is particularly useful as it fades if the blood pressure falls. (The carotid pulse is less satisfactory since it can be felt at low blood pressures and finger pressure in the baroreceptors of the carotid body may produce a fall of blood pressure.)
3. Be aware of the depth of anaesthesia.
4. Tell the dentist immediately a problem occurs or is foreseen.

For his part the dental surgeon should:

1. Be aware of the anaesthetist's *modus operandi*.
2. Be aware of the risk of oral contents interfering with the airway.
3. Co-operate in protecting the airways both with adequate packing of the oropharynx and with lower jaw support when feasible.
4. Tell the anaesthetist should any operative problem occur.

Despite all precautions, problems do occasionally arise. There is little doubt that their frequency depends on the training and experience of the 'team'.

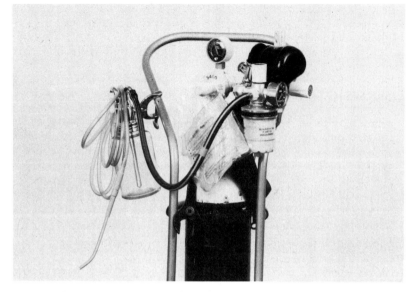

Fig. 8.1. A reserve oxygen supply. It has the advantage of also providing a reserve suction supply which although not powerful is not dependent on electric power.

SOLVING PROBLEMS

When problems do occur, solving them depends on (1) diagnosis and (2) treatment.

There are several different areas that need consideration, but without doubt maintaining respiratory and cardiovascular function is of fundamental importance.

Maintenance of Respiratory Function

Difficulties in respiration are usually a result of airway obstruction due to:

1. Anatomical variations (a large tongue, retrognathic mandible, enlarged adenoids and tonsils etc.).
2. Failure to maintain the airway (opening too wide, applying backward pressure during extraction, having the head flexed, failing to protrude the mandible, poor packing of the mouth etc.).
3. Pathological problems (upper respiratory tract infection, blocked nasal airways, adenoiditis etc.).
4. Laryngeal spasm (due to blood, saliva, mucus, pus, vomit, foreign bodies etc. touching the cords).
5. Obstruction below the vocal cords (inhaled foreign body, bronchospasm etc.).

COMPLICATIONS AND EMERGENCIES

Respiratory function can be observed by watching the movement of the anaesthetic reservoir bag and ensuring its movements are co-ordinated with the patient's chest movements. (A bag can be made to simulate normal respiration simply by repeatedly making and breaking the seal on the mask.) Audible expiratory valves provide another useful monitor but these are not infallible. If a patient is genuinely obstructed 'paradoxical' (see-saw) breathing often develops, resulting from the hard downward pull of the diaphragm, against an upper respiratory obstruction. (Sinking of the chest and protrusion of the abdomen with minimal air/gas intake results in the up and down see-saw action of the chest and abdomen (*Fig. 3.7*)).

If the obstruction is at the larynx it is usually but not always audible (as opposed to silent). When inspiration is attempted a high pitched whine may be heard. As the obstruction lessens, the pitch of the note decreases but in either case it should be treated as a serious complication. Even more serious is the total obstruction caused by tight contraction of the vocal cords (silent obstruction) as this can occur without warning and quickly leads on to cardiovascular collapse. None of these complications should be confused with the breath holding which may occur in Stage II, either during induction, or during a poorly maintained anaesthetic, when some mouth breathing has occurred and the depth of anaesthesia lightened. Movements of the limbs are usually seen during this condition and any laryngeal noises tend to be expiratory (phonation), caused by the patient trying to object vocally. The patient's colour usually remains good and providing the airway is kept patent, they will breathe again when the partial pressure of the blood carbon dioxide builds up sufficiently. Such is *not* the case with genuine obstruction which requires quick and accurate diagnosis as to its cause. Anatomical variations can frequently be corrected by protruding the mandible with firm pressure on the posterior border of the ramus of the jaw. It is important to ensure that the occlusion is not locked, particularly in patients with deep overbites. The Class II, Division 2 occlusion can present extreme difficulties in protruding the mandible and it is important to open the jaw before attempting to apply too much pressure. Patients who are obese or those with retrognathic mandibles also require careful management and sound technique to correct simple obstruction. Those with large tongues may prove difficult as Stage III anaesthesia occurs and the use of an oral airway to deepen the plane of anaesthesia may be indicated, when it is often easier to maintain a satisfactory airway.

Some of the other anatomical and operative complications have already been dealt with. Over-ambitious opening of the mouth, incorrect use of force in removing mandibular (or even maxillary teeth), incorrect positioning of the head and poor mouth packing are usually easily corrected. In some patients enlarged adenoids or small nasal polyps occasionally prevent the establishing of a good nasal airway. While it is occasionally possible to complete a very short procedure with mouth-breathing being allowed it is usually totally unsatisfactory. Nasal airways can be used but they are not without their problems. The soft, flanged rubber nasal airways (e.g. the Bardex or Goldman) are probably the safest and most suitable. These are available in a variety of sizes and usually numbered in a way which is inversely proportional to their diameter and length. In principle they support a clear nasal passage and rest posteriorly in the naso-pharynx. Before inserting them a sufficient depth of anaesthesia is required and after lubricating them with a sterile gel they should be gently passed into one of the nostrils. The right nostril is commonly considered better, but if any frank obstruction is encountered the left side should be attempted. The degree of obstruction is usually related to the deviation of the nasal septum. The suggestion is that it more commonly deviates to the left side in the posterior nasal passages, making the right side relatively larger. In no circumstances should airways be forced into position as the last thing wanted at this stage is mucosal bleeding.

There are different ways of classifying airway obstruction. They may be pathologically sub-divided or anatomically sub-divided. Anatomical sub-division can be related to:

1. Blockage in the lumen.
2. Blockage in the wall.
3. Pressure external to the wall.

Alternatively, the various levels of obstruction from the nasal apertures down to the alveoli form a suitable basis on which to examine some of the common problems affecting anaesthesia.

Blockage of the lumen of the air passages is the most common type of obstruction. If this is in the nose a nasal airway may be useful in overcoming minor secretions, but it may prove unsuitable for physical blockages, such as could be caused by nasal polyps (or even tumours). As well as the problems of potential breathing, airways which are too short may be ineffective whilst those which are too long can end up either in the oesophagus or on the back of the tongue, further occluding the airway. They may even on occasion reach the larynx when they could provoke a dangerous laryngospasm.

In addition to nasal obstruction it is possible to block the airway in the mouth or pharynx. This is usually a result of either failing to position the pack correctly in relation to the tongue and soft palate, or due to the operator pushing his fingers into the lingual sulcus, usually in supporting the sockets of the posterior tooth he is extracting. Since two objects cannot occupy the same space at the same time, this practice frequently results in the tongue being forced backwards and blocking the tracheal opening. It should, however, be relatively easy to correct mechanical obstruction of this type, whereas laryngeal obstruction is more serious since it is much harder to correct.

The reflex activity of the larynx is preserved until an extremely deep plane of anaesthesia is achieved. This should never occur in outpatient dental anaesthesia, since maintenance of the body's own protective mechanisms is highly desirable. Foreign matter touching the vocal cords (be it mucus, blood, pus, vomit or whatever) can stimulate the larynx into a tight contraction known as laryngeal spasm or stridor. Any sound produced will be high pitched and audible during attempted inspiration. It should be treated immediately by increasing the oxygen content of the gases (to 100% in severe spasm), sucking out any contents of the mouth or pharynx and posturing the head to avoid further contamination of the cords. In practice the lateral position with the head tilted down is the safest posture to adopt since it not only protects the airway but gives support to the cardiovascular system. The vast majority of spasms will spontaneously relax if these simple corrective measures are followed and there is little place in outpatient practice for attempting an intubation, giving muscle relaxants or trying a tracheostomy. Such measures are rarely employed despite their theoretical necessity. If the patient's condition does not spontaneously improve the simplest and safest technique to attempt is a crico-thyrotomy (coniotomy) (*Fig.* 8.2). The neck is extended and a crico-thyroid needle inserted through or just below the crico-thyroid membrane. Even the insertion of a 14G intravenous cannula will allow enough air intake to be life-saving until help can be summoned,

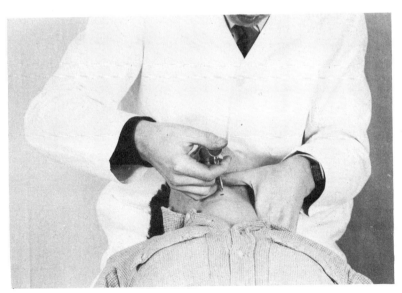

Fig. 8.2. Cricothyrotomy with a tracheotome. The crico-thyroid membrane is marked, the neck extended and the skin tensed before insertion (cf. *Fig.* 3.9). Penetration of the trachea will be rendered easier by making a small skin incision prior to insertion.

particularly if it can be connected up to oxygen under some pressure (*Fig. 3.9*). It should be stressed that careless suction may in fact initiate or aggravate a laryngeal spasm and that careful use of rounded smooth suckers is essential. The high volume plastic suckers are preferred (e.g. the Yankauer) but metal ones may be satisfactory. Detachable sucker ends should not be used.

Foreign bodies such as teeth, roots or fragments of tissue should never escape behind the pack. In the event of such an accident the head should be positioned to protect the airway before any attempt to recover it is made. While it is very tempting to put one's fingers in the mouth and try and catch the offending item, the anatomy is such that it is likely to slide away into the pharynx or larynx. Once the patient is in the head-down lateral position, it is relatively easy to recover it with the help of a laryngoscope and Magill's forceps or even tweezers.

In the unfortunate event of the item disappearing from sight, it is essential to locate it postoperatively by the use of chest and abdomen radiographs. If it has fallen past the cords into the trachea, it usually drops into the right bronchus. From there it can only be recovered by bronchoscopy but if this is performed promptly the patient is unlikely to suffer any long term sequelae. (The same may not be true of the dentist!) Teeth or roots in the stomach will normally pass uneventfully through the alimentary canal. Rarely a tooth may lodge between the cords and while it may be possible to recover it with Magill's forceps (*Fig. 7.4*), this is one instance where bypassing the cords is beneficial, by means of a cricothyrotomy rather than attempted tracheostomy.

The final type of obstruction occurs at a level below the vocal cords, usually in the bronchi. This may be due to excessive bronchial secretions, bronchiectasis, asthmatic attack or bronchospasm. It is usually a sub-total obstruction of varying degree which should be treated with increased oxygenation. In the outpatient situation the anaesthetic should be abandoned and careful recovery supervised. Specialist treatment may involve the use of broncho-dilators such as salbutamol or anti-asthmatic drugs such as aminophylline. The use of these and other 'emergency' drugs is discussed later, but there should be little place for them in the dental surgery.

Protection of the airway is the most vital part of any complication and occasional adverse drug reactions may cause apnoea (absence of breathing). This is most likely to be encountered with diazepam, particularly if analgesic supplements have also been administered. It is also a recognized side-effect of fentanyl. In such patients the respiratory receptors and centre appear depressed and the patient, while looking alert and conscious, gradually gets progressively cyanosed. Such patients usually respond to requests to breathe but if they do not, it is easy to ventilate them with oxygen or with air using an Ambu-bag (*Fig. 8.3*). It should be stressed here that some reserve supply of oxygen which can be admini-

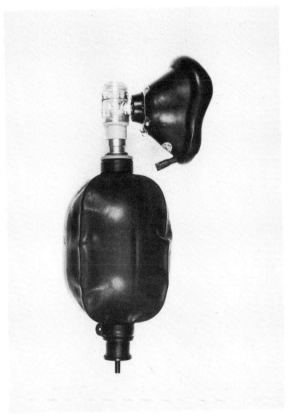

Fig. 8.3. The Ambu-bag. It is self-inflating and can be connected to an oxygen supply if one is available.

stered under positive pressure is regarded as essential equipment in the dental surgery. Providing the patient is immediately ventilated they recover with a remarkable rapidity. Failure to notice the deterioration in the patient's colour has potentially serious consequences since absence of sufficient oxygenated blood reaching the brain for more than a short period of time will result not only in cardiac arrest, but in potential permanent brain damage.

Maintenance of Cardiovascular Function

In the dental surgery the procedure for treatment of a cardiac arrest needs to be predetermined, practised and efficient. It is useless going out to dial

999 while the patient is arrested. It is therefore suggested that the following course of treatment is followed:
1. Establish that cardiac arrest has occurred.
2. Get nurse/receptionist to dial 999. Summon useful help. Note the exact time.
3. Treat the arrest by:
    a. Ventilating patient.
    b. External cardiac massage (*Fig.* 8.4).

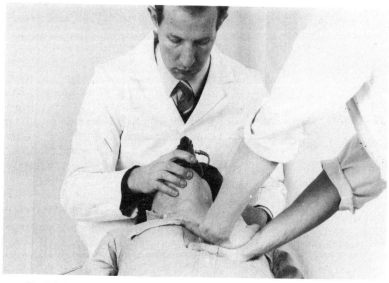

Fig. 8.4. Artificial ventilation and external cardiac massage. Pressure should be applied to the base of the sternum to compress the heart between it and the spine.

The diagnosis of cardiac arrest is not as easy as it sounds. Many cases of fainting or respiratory arrest have been treated over-enthusiastically and fractured ribs are not pleasant! Conversely failure to recognize the possibility of arrest or delaying treatment until all signs of arrest are present may prove fatal. The three classic signs of a cardiac arrest are absence of pulse, ashen-grey appearance of the skin and fixed dilatation of the pupils. The difficulties of these signs lie in the fact that they can easily be camouflaged. Following a respiratory arrest for instance the pulse quickly weakens and may be found absent by an inexperienced practitioner. Similarly the change in skin colour is as dependent on the quantity of haemoglobin in the blood as it is on the actual blood flow. The ashen-grey appearance is a combination of peripheral vaso-constriction and cyanosis, the latter being caused by the presence of at least 5 g deoxygenated haemoglobin per 100 ml blood. The fixed dilated pupil is also a late sign of cardiac arrest and should not be awaited before treatment is commenced.

If a cardiac arrest is suspected, the patient should be ventilated with oxygen for 10–15 s, having checked the patency of the upper airway. In the case of respiratory arrest this would produce an immediate improvement in the patient's colour and of the pulse strength. In the case of cardiac arrest the patient's colour continues to deteriorate. External cardiac massage should be started immediately. For this the patient should be on a flat, rigid surface. The vast majority of fully reclined dental chairs are suitable for this purpose but the more luxuriously padded chairs may not provide enough support. The most satisfactory position from which to work is with the team leader ventilating the patient from the 12 o'clock position. The assistant is positioned at 3 o'clock and uses both hands on top of each other to apply firm downward pressure to the base of the sternum. The heart is then compressed between the sternum and the vertebrae and blood is expelled into the peripheral circulation. Opinions vary as to the ratio of compressions/ventilations but it should not exceed 6:1. External cardiac massage and intermittent ventilation can be kept up almost indefinitely until help arrives. It may not result in the heart starting to beat spontaneously but it can prevent the brain being totally starved of the oxygen it needs to survive. The reason that the heart is unlikely to restart is due to the development of other factors, caused by the arrest itself. In itself, this is a detailed subject and it is well covered in the relevant textbooks. In particular, however, the build up of carbon dioxide results in a fall in the blood pH due to the build up of carbonic acid, a condition known as respiratory acidosis, which is corrected with artificial ventilation. The severe metabolic acidosis resulting from the lack of tissue perfusion will require intravenous sodium bicarbonate for correction. The unbalanced relationship between respiration and metabolism also leads to a fall in the value of the ionized calcium fraction in the blood. The effect of this is to induce tetany in skeletal muscle; in cardiac muscle it may result in decreased contractile strength. The later consequences of this are ventricular fibrillation and decreased chances of resuscitation.

Diuretics may well be needed after a prolonged arrest coupled with intravenous fluids to balance the shift that occurs from intracellular to extracellular fluid. The other ionic constituents of the blood (electrolytes) also become unbalanced but these can, on the whole be corrected later. Cardiac arrest is a useful term since it describes the clinical condition of the patient. It is not, however, a diagnosis on which to base detailed treatment. The two common causes of cardiac arrest are asystole (where the heart literally stops) and ventricular fibrillation (where the heart is subjected to excess unco-ordinated electrical activity). Whereas intravenous adrenaline may cure asystole it will aggravate ventricular fibrillation.

Conversely giving an electric shock to defibrillate a patient with asystole is useless and potentially harmful. The differential diagnosis of these conditions can only be made with the use of an electrocardiogram (ECG). For these reasons management of cardiac arrest in the dental surgery is best restricted to the simple measures outlined above.

Successful external cardiac massage is recognized by the reversal of the original factors, *viz.* the skin colour improves, the pulse is palpable in time with each compression and the pupil size diminishes. However, massage should be continued even if the only sign of success is a coincidental carotid pulse until expert care is available. In the event of failure of the reserve oxygen, mouth-to-mouth or mouth-to-nose breathing should be used. The techniques for this can be found in all the textbooks on first-aid or resuscitation. Cardiac and respiratory arrest are not the only complications of general anaesthesia.

Hypertension, Hypotension and Fainting

The past 10 years has seen a marked shift in anaesthetic opinion away from the seated position to the supine or Trendelenberg position. The reason for this is that there is some evidence to suggest that significant falls of blood pressure may occur during anaesthesia without any obvious clinical signs. Some fall in blood pressure would be expected during anaesthesia since the stress generated by the proposed operation is likely to cause an initial rise which is then relieved. Equally many of the anaesthetic agents in use are known to induce falls of blood pressure. The risk of marked vaso-vagal activity has received much attention and the consequence has been to reject the seated position. The disadvantage of this (not often mentioned by its proponents) is that the degree of natural airway protection is much less in the supine position. Even in the supine position falls in blood pressure can occur, be they vaso-vagal or due to a hypotensive reactions. The phenothiazines are said to induce hypotension and since these may on occasion be used for treating hay fever, it is well to be cautious of people with allergic histories—particularly if the pollen count is high and the weather hot! In all cases the blood supply to the brain must be maintained at a satisfactory level. To achieve this the legs should be raised and the head tilted down. Atropine 0·6 mg given intravenously is potentially useful and unlikely to be harmful. The anticholinergic effects of atropine depress vagal activity and therefore lead to an increased heart rate. If excess fluid loss is suspected (for example as a result of excessive bleeding) a drip, preferably of balanced electrolytes should be established.

Hypertension may occur as a result of acidosis following inadequate gas exchange. In such cases improving the breathing, using positive pressure ventilation if necessary, will quickly correct matters. In others, however, the rise in blood pressure may be due to the stimulus of surgery when the patient is inadequately anaesthetized. This is simply corrected by deepening the plane of anaesthesia, if the surgery is to continue for any length of time. Occasionally hypertension can occur as a drug interaction with patients who are taking tricyclic antidepressants or monoamine oxidase inhibitors. In such patients the effect of catecholamines (adrenaline-type drugs) is potentiated and serious hypertension can result. In such cases effective treatment can only be achieved by abandoning the anaesthetic and giving a β-blocking agent such as propranolol.

Patients with pre-existent hypertension are far more susceptible to changes in blood pressure in either direction. The reason for this is that hypertension usually represents a failure of the vessels to compensate for the normal changes of blood pressure produced in systole and diastole. Any additional factor affecting the cardiac output, be it hypertensive or hypotensive therefore has an amplified effect. The recognition of such blood pressure changes is not always easy and the only conclusive proof is provided by monitoring it. Some of the modern electronic aids with bleeps, flashing lights and digital read-outs make this a very simple procedure, and if there is any doubt about the patient's preoperative state the blood pressure should be checked. Blood pressure is a function of cardiac output and peripheral resistance, so in either area problems may occur; their treatment is a matter for specialists.

Vomiting

Vomiting and regurgitation are much more commonly observed in the outpatient situation than in the hospitalized patient. This is in part due to the role of preoperative medication and partly to the incidence being lower with the intravenous agents compared with the inhalational ones. Though it can occur during induction or maintenance of anaesthesia (either light or fluctuating), it is usually seen during recovery. It is also a problem in outpatient anaesthesia as the anaesthetist has to rely on the word of the patient (or parent) that no food or drink has been consumed. Most patients do this reliably, but some deliberately conceal the truth or are deceived by their children. The presence of pain can cause delayed emptying of gastric contents but the 6 h rule is normally safe.

Vomiting, unlike regurgitation which is passive, is a result of reflex activity from the medulla through to the vagus nerve. The stimulus acts on the stomach, diaphragm, larynx and respiratory muscles. Theoretically, the risk of aspirating after vomiting is low since the laryngeal reflexes must still be present, but in practice it does happen occasionally when the patient is hypoxic and gasps for air. Regurgitation, though less common, is more serious since there is a serious risk of inhalation. Again the head-down lateral position is the most effective for relieving problems and the pharynx can then be cleared mechanically with effective suction. Any vomit inhaled into the trachea should be aspirated immediately using a laryngoscope to establish direct vision. Prevention of regurgitation is possible by applying firm backward pressure on the cricoid cartilage. This does not compromise the airway when carried out correctly, but permits occlusion of the oesophagus, thus minimizing the risks of further regurgitation and inhalation.

If sufficient vomit is inhaled there is a risk of Mendelson's syndrome—an acute bronchospasm (caused by the low pH of the acidic vomit) which is followed by circulatory collapse. This should be treated immediately with intravenous hydrocortisone 100 mg and an anti-bronchospasm agent such as aminophylline. One hundred per cent oxygen should be given with positive pressure ventilation. Even quickly corrected as many as 20% of patients so afflicted may subsequently die. The long-term risk of patients less severely afflicted is the development of pneumonitis and bronchitis.

Overdosage and Supersensitivity

The level of response to any drug is related to many different factors, the individual patient being the most important, yet unfortunately, the least controllable of these. Within the patient himself the effect of a drug is dependent on body weight, emotional state, metabolic rate, general health, presence of pain and other factors. Most drugs have a wide safety margin but this is no excuse for careless practice since once an intravenous agent has been injected there is no way it can be removed again! Many of the problems associated with the intravenous agents were discussed in Chapter 2 but some points require reiteration.

Thiopentone/Methohexitone

Both these short acting intravenous barbiturates are commonly used, though methohexitone is more frequently used in outpatient practice, due to its shorter action and its less painful qualities when injected. The consequences of intra-arterial injection are discussed later.

Overdosage with short-acting barbiturates can lead to respiratory and circulatory collapse. It usually occurs in two situations; the first is an initial dose too large for the patient and the second is using incremental techniques with too large repeat doses. In either case the general principles for resuscitation outlined in the earlier part of this chapter should be followed, with particular care to provide adequate gaseous exchange.

Althesin

This short-acting double steroid anaesthetic has been reported on several occasions to cause an anaphylactic type of collapse. It is probably due to the solvent, Cremophor EL which was used with propanidid and even with diazepam. Treatment of the collapse is to give oxygen, intravenous hydrocortisone 100 mg and antihistamines. The use of subcutaneous adrenaline and intravenous fluid support therapy may also be considered.

Diazepam

Diazepam has wide safety margins but does occasionally result in apnoea and deep sleep. Occasionally patients may even be totally anaesthetized. In all such cases the protection of the airway and the support of respiratory function is essential. The other general complication of higher doses is the slow half-life of its active metabolites which may result in patients feeling a little remote for up to 5 days. The local complications of diazepam injections are discussed later.

Allergy, Anaphylaxis and Hypersensitivity

The possibility of stimulating an allergic type reaction is present with every drug, though with some the incidence is higher. The range of presentations of such reactions can be extremely varied from a slight skin rash to anaphylactic collapse. The former is extremely irritating, the latter potentially fatal within minutes. The risk of this is greatest in patients with an 'allergic' history (which should be known). Certain classes of drugs are also known to have a greater risk of inducing anaphylaxis. Amongst these penicillin is most commonly known, but the solvent Cremophor-EL (present in both Althesin and propanidid) is not unusual in causing it.

The symptoms of anaphylaxis are extremely variable. A loss of consciousness due to circulatory collapse may be accompanied by bronchospasm, peripheral oedema, nausea, sweating and anything from a minimal erythematous skin rash to a total erythema.

The treatment of anaphylaxis is somewhat controversial. Certain measures would have universal acceptance and these include:
1. Lying the patient head down and legs raised.
2. Administering 100% oxygen.
3. Intravenous administration of hydrocortisone 100 mg and intravenous anti-histamines (e.g. promethazine 25–50 mg).

The anti-histamines are seldom as effective in practice as they are in theory, possibly because the true anaphylaxis is not mediated by histamine release. The administration of adrenaline (1 : 1000) by subcutaneous or intramuscular injection is contentious. Some would argue it to be lifesaving; others that it is ineffective and potentially adds further complications. Similarly treating bronchospasm with aminophylline may or may not be effective. The problem with all these aspects of treatment is the rarity with which complications are encountered. Consequently simple measures designed to protect the circulation and its oxygenation have much to commend them.

The possibility of supervening cardiac arrest must be borne in mind and treated immediately if the need arises.

Atypical Reactions

The variations of individual reaction to each anaesthetic is extreme. Atypical reactions may be related to various aspects of the patient's state or metabolism. These may be frank pathologies or no more than an extension of the usually considered normal limit. In the former category malignant hyperthermia (hyperpyrexia) is a fairly rare reaction. As the name suggests it is characterized by a progressive rise in body temperature usually with other signs of increased metabolic activity such as increased muscular tone. It has been suggested that some sort of sensitization may be necessary but this should not be assumed. Halothane, thiopentone and suxamethonium have all been implicated but it may be that no agent is exempt from the possibility of causing malignant hyperthermia. It should be treated by administering pure oxygen, intravenous dantrolene and active cooling, particularly of the head and neck region, though immediate admission to hospital should be arranged.

A non-pathological example of an atypical reaction is the delayed recovery. While this may be a consequence of overdosage or supersensitivity there are instances when neither seems apparent and yet patients do not regain consciousness in a reasonable time. While this may be worrying it is not serious providing due consideration is given to the state of the respiration and circulation. If both can be shown to be satisfactory it is usually only a matter of time before the patient recovers.

This is not the case in the few patients who have a hereditary deficiency of pseudo-choline esterase, the enzyme which metabolizes suxamethonium. In such patients the return of spontaneous respiration (after the administration of suxamethonium) may be delayed for periods of up to 48 h, though 1–12 h is more usual. Continuous ventilation with fairly deep sedation is needed to protect the blood oxygenation and to alleviate the distress caused by being conscious but unable to breathe or move. Since this enzyme deficiency has a hereditary element the relatives of any patient detected should be fully investigated. It hardly needs saying that pseudo-choline esterase deficient patients should not be given suxamethonium.

LOCAL COMPLICATIONS

The use of sound venepuncture technique should minimize or obviate most of the possible complications. The possibility of extravenous injection is perhaps the most common complication. It may occur as a result of not penetrating the lumen of the vein completely (or even partially) or as a result of tissuing (allowing the needle to pass out into the tissues during the course of an injection). Small quantities of extravenous deposits will usually disperse freely and uneventfully, though an acute inflammatory reaction may ensue. Larger volumes may require firm massaging to disperse them and some would suggest the administration of vasodilators and the enzyme hyaluronidase. The aim of treatment is to encourage the rapid uptake into the blood stream so that delayed effects of the agent get little chance to occur.

Intra-arterial injection should be impossible if the correct techniques are used. Brachial artery spasm is a dangerous condition characterized by an intense burning pain radiating from the site of injection *down* the arm. The skin blanches and the radial and ulnar pulses weaken to the point of absence. Unless quickly treated, the static blood coagulates causing thrombosis which subsequently leads to gangrene. The only treatment for this is amputation—more than a little unfortunate if the intra-arterial injection was supposedly to relieve toothache! It should have been avoided:

1. By not injecting medial to the biceps tendon.
2. By aspirating and observing the unusual redness of the blood.
3. By injecting only a minimal quantity and asking if pain was felt. The affirmative answer and the pain location are diagnostic.

Treatment is difficult. If possible the needle is left in position so that it can be used to administer drugs into the artery. Procaine 1% is usually advised since it is a vasodilator as well as a local analgesic. The patient should be immediately referred to hospital where various surgical techniques or brachial plexus block may be possible alternatives if the spasm has not resolved.

Good intravenous injections have little morbidity but the risk of venous thrombosis following intravenous diazepam is well known. This risk can of course be minimized with the emulsion and with careful techniques, but even so an occasional incident results. Various methods have been tried to disperse thromboses, from topical creams to anticoagulants. There can be little doubt that they usually resolve in time but the condition can be painful and if resolution does not occur in 10–14 days, patients should be referred to their medical practitioners.

Injuries caused during treatment are usually a result of faulty procedure. The soft tissues of the face are easily traumatized, the lower lip being at particular risk. If injuries do occur they should be examined and treated while the patient is asleep. They, or their parents, should then be told what has happened without concealing the facts. Deceitful statements such as 'she bit her lip' etc. merely open the way for legal action on two fronts rather than one. An honest apology on the other hand is nearly always accepted without further action. Similarly if wrong teeth are removed or displaced, gingiva torn, work incompleted etc. this should also be reported.

The occurrence of temporomandibular joint dislocation is rare and should be recognized before the patient's recovery. Relocating the temporomandibular joint is certainly an easier procedure under a general anaesthetic. It should be accomplished by pushing the jaw firmly downwards and backwards from the region of the molar teeth. The easiest way to achieve this is to use the external oblique ridge of the mandible as this allows good access and avoids trauma to the surgeon if the jaw-closing reflex is elicited.

Fractures of the jaw are fortunately rare complications of extractions. The patient should normally be woken and fully assessed to confirm the diagnosis—even if it is (or appears) obvious—before any definitive treatment is arranged.

Other injuries under anaesthetic should be assessed while the patient is still anaesthetized and where practical, repair of the damage should be made at this time.

The basis of all good anaesthesia is careful assessment, sound knowledge and safe practice. It is hoped that in reading this text, the student may feel more confident in approaching his clinical training in anaesthesia and sedation, and that he may feel more inspired to look into the more advanced textbooks to follow up lines of thought which have been outside the scope of this book.

BIBLIOGRAPHY

Atkinson R. S., Rushman G. B. and Lee J. A. (1982) *A Synopsis of Anaesthesia*, 9th ed. Bristol, Wright.

Comroe J. H. (1974) *Physiology of Respiration: An Introductory Text*. Chicago, Year Book.

Kelman G. R. (1977) *Applied Cardiovascular Physiology*, 2nd ed. Sevenoaks, Butterworths.

Langa H. (1976) *Relative Analgesia in Dental Practice*. Philadelphia, Saunders.

Robinson R. and Stott R. (1980) *Medical Emergencies and Management*, 3rd ed. London, Heinemann.

Vickers M. D., Wood-Smith F. G. and Stewart H. C. (1978) *Drugs in Anaesthetic Practice*, 5th ed. Sevenoaks, Butterworths.

INDEX

Bold type indicates the principal references.

abscess, dental, 6
acetyl choline, 124
acetyl choline esterase, 37, 126
acidaemia, 9
acidosis, 137
acromegaly, 118
adenosine triphosphate (ATP), 29
adrenal gland, 8
adrenaline
  in emergency, 129, 137, 141
  endogenous, 25
  exogenous, 26, 52
age, relationship to anaesthesia, 3
air, alveolar, 29
airway
  anatomy of, 44
  control of, 13, 56, 91, 99, 130, 138
  patency, 15
airway obstruction, **44ff**
  causes of, 6, 11, 58
  classification of, 132
  complications of, 121
  effects of, 18, 131
  management of, **50**
  signs of, **47ff**, 58
  with packs, 53
alcohol, 14, 79, 82, 88, 95
alcuronium, 126
alkalaemia, 9
allergy, 12, 88, 138, **141**
alphadolone, *see* Althesin
alphaxolone, *see* Althesin
Althesin, 36, **88**, 99, 140
alveolus, 19, 21
Ambu-bag, 134–5
aminophylline, 52, 129, 134
amnesia, 37, 68
anaemia, 7, 8
anaesthesia
  in asthmatics, 25
  in children, 3, 22, 37, 115, 122
  complications, of, **128**, 142
  depth of, 53
  endotracheal, **107**
  general, 1
  induction of, **38**
  inhalational, **16ff**
  instructions for, 13, 36
  intravenous, **79ff**
  limitations of, 10
  local, *see* Local anaesthesia

anaesthesia (*cont.*)
  maintenance of, **53**
  outpatient, 1, 13, 90
  positions of, **40ff**
  preparation for, **13ff**
  recovery from, *see* Recovery
  stages of, 38, 70, 86
  trends in, 102, 138
anaesthetic
  agents, 79
  circuits, **66**
  inhalational, 84
  local, 12, 26
  machines, 23, **59ff**
  potency, 21
analgesia, 39, 69, *see also* Relative
    analgesia
anaphylaxis, 88, 141
angina, 5
ankylosing spondylitis, 118
ante-cubital fossa, **81**
anticoagulant, 11, 12
anticonvulsant, 10
antidepressant, 11
anti-emetic, 96
antihistimine, 105, 141
antisialogogue, **105**, 121
anxiety, 4, 13
apnoea
  during anaesthesia, 39, 86, 122
  with diazepam, 100, 134, 141
  with fentanyl, 134
  see also Respiratory depression
arrhythmias, *see* Cardiac arrhythmias
artery
  brachial, 82, 83, 143
  coronary, 25
  injection into, 143
aspiration, 107, 139
asthma, 134
asystole, 124, 137
ataraxia, 73
atlanto-occipital joint, 50, 118
atracurium, 126
atropine, 125, 129, 138

back, disorders of, 10
Bain circuit, 66
barbiturates, **34ff**, 96

INDEX

Bardex, see Nasal airways
baroreceptors, 129
benzodiazepines, 37, 95, 102
biceps, see Tendon
bladder, control of, 14
β-blocker, 139
blood
 clotting of, 8
 disorders of, 7, 8, 106
 electrolytes, 137
 flow, 25
 gas distribution coefficient, 19ff, see also relevant gases and agents
 gas exchange, 8
 loss, 8
 pH, 17, 137
 solubility, 19
 sugar, 8
 volume, 4, 7
blood pressure, **5**
 control of, 9, 90
 lowered, 26, 27, 53, 138
 raised, 6, 12, 49
blood-brain barrier, 17
Bodok seal, 60, 61
Boyle machine, see Anaesthetic machines
brachial plexus, 143
bradycardia, 9, 125, 127
brain
 damage to, 6, 41, 122, 135
 function of, 10
 stem, 18
breathing, see Ventilation
bronchiectasis, 134
bronchiole, 25
bronchitis, 6, 17, 73, 140
bronchoconstriction, 25
bronchodilator, see Salbutamol
bronchospasm, 6, 36, 134, 140
bronchus, 19
buffer, 17
burns, 124
butterfly needle, 84, 85

calcium gluconate, 129
calcium, ionized, 137
carbon dioxide
 effects of, **25ff**
 partial pressure, 25
 retention of, 108
carbonic acid, 17, 137
cardiac arrest, 22, 28, 29, 50, **135ff**
cardiac arrhythmias, 26, 38, 50, 52, 108

cardiac output, 5, 20, 33, 36, 53, 139
cardiac rhythm, 24
cardiovascular system
 collapse of, 81, 131, 140
 depression of, 26, 35, 36
 disorders of, 5ff, 11
 maintenance of, **135ff**
 physiology of, 20ff
 see also Blood pressure and cardiac
Carotid body, 17
catecholamines
 endogenous, 22, 25, 28, 49, 108
 exogenous, 11
 see also Adrenaline
cerebral blood flow, 25
cerebrospinal fluid, 17
cervical spine, 118
chemoreceptors, 17
chloral hydrate, 97
chloroform, 22, 28, 29, 38
chlorpheniramine, 129
cholinesterase
 see Acetylcholinesterase
 see pseudo-Cholinestarase
Christmas disease, 12
circuits, see Anaesthetic circuits
circulation, see Cardiovascular system
claudication, intermittent, 5
colour coding, 60
coniotomy, see Cricothyrotomy
continuous flow, see Equipment
Cordus, Valerius, 28
coughing, 6, 26
Coulton, Quincy, 22
coumarin, 97
Cremophor EL, 36, 88, 141
cricoid, 140
cricothyrotomy, 52, **133**
cuffs, see Endotracheal tubes
curare, 27, 125
cyanosis, 7, 100
 causes of, 49, 85, 134
 observation of, 5, 14, 137
cyclopropane, 22
cylinders, gas, 16, 60
 key for, 64

dacuronium, 126
Dalton's Law, 21, 25, 29
Davy, Humphry, 22
dead space, 19
death, 8, 12, 13, 28
dehydration, 7
demand flow, 70

146

INDEX

depression, 11
desmethyldiazepine, 100
dextrose, 129
diabetes, 8, 9
diaphragm, 18
diazepam, 37, 90, 134
  emulsion, 102
  in emergency, 129
  intravenous, **99**
  oral, **95**
  premedication, 104
diffusion hypoxia, *see* Hypoxia
dislocation, of jaw, 143
diuretics, 137
Down's syndrome, 11
droperidol, 101
drugs
  activity of, 32–4
  addiction to, 11
  binding of, 32
  doses of, 91
  ionization of, 32, 33
  in plasma, 32
  problems with, 11, 140
  redistribution of, 32ff, 80, 85
  taking of, 10
Drummond-Jackson, 92, 98
dystrophia myotonica, 124

electrocardiogram, 5, 138
electroencephalogram, 27
electrolytes, 9
electrophoresis, 8
embolism, 79
emergency, **128ff**
emotions, 17
emphysema, 73
endotracheal anaesthesia, **107ff**
  complications, 120
  contra-indications, 108
  equipment for, 109
  indications, 107
  techniques, 109
  types, 107
endotracheal tubes, 107, **110**, 129
  cuffs of, 110, 111
epilepsy, 10
epistaxis, 50
equipment
  for anaesthesia, 50
  for analgesia, **70**
  checking of, 72
  emergency, 129

escorts, 14
esters, 36
ether, 19, 26, 28, 38
  halogenated, 26, 27
ethyl chloride, 21, 28, 29, 38
etomidate, 36, 89
eugenol, 36, 89
euphoria, 24, 43, 104
excretion, 9, 33, 80
expiration, *see* Ventilation
explosive, 28
extraction
  technique, 56
  wrong, 143
extubation, **119**, 122
eyelash reflex, 39, 53, 91

fail-safe mechanism, 65
fainting, 41, 136, 138
fat, 34, 36
fazadinium, 126
fear, 13
fentanyl, **101**, 125, 134
fibrillation
  atrial, 9
  ventricular, 137
Fischer, Emil, 28
flowmeter, 20, 70, *see also* Rotameter
flow rates, 75
fluid loss, 138
fluoride ion, 27, 28
fractures, jaw, 144
fresh gas flow, 63
frusemide, 129

gag, 91, 129
galactosaemia, 9
gas
  exchange, 49
  laughing, 24
gastric juices, 13
giggles, 76
glyceryl trinitrate, 5
Goldman
  airway, 132
  vaporizer, 64–5
Griffiths, 125
Guedel, 38

hand, veins of, 81
haematology, *see* Blood

147

INDEX

haemoglobin, 7, **29**ff
  dissociation, 29
  sickled, 7
haemolysis, 7
haemophilia, 8, 12
halothane, 20, 21, **24**ff, 125, 142
  concentrations, 53
  history, 38
  phamacology, 18
  repeated doses, 25
  toxicity of, 9, 52
headache, 80
heart murmur, *see* Cardiovascular system
heart rate, 49, *see also* Bradycardia, Tachycardia
hiccuping, 86, 87
hospital, treatment in, 9
hydrocortisone, 129, 140, 141
hydrogen ion, 17, *see also* Blood pH
hyoscine, 98
hypercapnoea, 49
hyperpyrexia *see* Malignant hyperpyrexia
hypersensitivity, *see* Allergy
hypertension, *see* Blood pressure
hyperthyroidism, *see* Thyroid
hypnosedatives, 103, **104**
hypnosis, 73, 74
hypocapnoea, 27
hypotension, *see* Blood pressure
hypothyroidism, *see* Thyroid
hypoxaemia, 26
hypoxia, 38, 49, 50, 99
  diffusion, 23, 26, 77, 119

incremental techniques, 80, 84, 86, 92, 98
induction, 36, **38**
inhalational anaesthesia, **38**ff
  agents in, 16
  pharmacology, **16**
inhalational sedation, **68**ff
injection
  fate of, 32
  technique, *see* Venepuncture
inspiration, *see* Ventilation
  peak flow rate, 50
instructions, anaesthetic, 14
intermittent positive pressure ventilation, 108
intravenous anaesthesia, **79**ff
  agents in, **30**ff
  indications for, 79
  onset of action, 32
  pharmacology of, 30
  recovery from, 34
  redistribution in, 33

intravenous cannulae, 129
intravenous sedation, **97**
introducer, 129
intubation *see also* Endotracheal anaesthesia
  failure of, 117
  nasal, 37, 109
  techniques, 109
ischaemia
  of brain, 41
  of leg, 5
  of myocardium, 6
isoflurane, **27**ff

Jorgensen, Niels, 98

ketamine, 37, 89, 99
kidney
  disorders of, 9
  toxic effects on, 28

labetalol, 90
Lack circuit, 67
lateral position, 58, 133
laughing gas, *see* Nitrous oxide
laryngeal obstruction, 46
laryngoscopes, **112**ff, 129, 134
laryngoscopy, 109, **115**
laryngospasm, 41, 51ff, 112
  iatrogenic, 134
  in respiratory disease, 6
  with enflurane, 26
  with obstruction, 46, 119, 130, 133
larynx, 19
  reflexes of, 132
  oedema of, 122
lethal dose (LD), 80
lignocaine, 116
lipid solubility, 21, 36
liver
  disorders of, 9
  drug metablism in, 32ff, 36
  halothane effects, 25
  toxic effects on, 28
local anaesthesia, 1, 4, 11, 12, 77
local complications (of anaesthesia), 142
Long, Crawford, 28
lorazepam, **95**
Ludwig's angina, 6

148

INDEX

Macintosh, Sir Robert, 112, 115
macroglossia, 118, 131
macrogol, see Cremophor
Magill circuit, 66
Magill forceps, 52, 113–4, 134
malaise, 10
malignant hyperpyrexia, 125, 142
malonic acid, 34
maple syrup disease, 9
Mendelson's syndrome, 46, 140
mental handicap, 2, 10, 11
mental illness, see Depression
mental retardation, 9
metabolic acidosis, 137
metabolic disorders, **8**
metabolic rate, 10
β-methasone, 128
methohexitone, **35**ff, 86, 98, 140
micrognathia, 118
midazolam, 37
minimal alveolar concentration (MAC), 21–7
minute volume, 19, 72
mongolism, see Down's syndrome
mono-amine oxidase inhibitors, 11
morphine, 103, 104
mortality, see Death
mouth, 19, 91
mucus, 6
multiple sclerosis, 10
muscle relaxants, 52, **122**ff
muscle tone, 10
muscles
  accessory, 18
  intercostal, 19
  relaxed, 21, 26
  of respiration, 17
  tone, 10
myasthenia gravis, 10
myocardial depression, 24, 26, 115
myocardial oxygen requirements, 25
myxoedema, see Thyroid

narcosis, 21, 89
narcotic, 18, 103
nasal airway, 45, 50, 129, 132
nasal obstruction, 44
nausea, 80
neck disorders, 11
needles, see Venepunture
neostigmine, 126
nerve
  intercostal, 18

nerve (*cont.*)
  median, 82, 83
  phrenic, 18
  toxic effects on, 28
nervous system, disorders of, 9
neuroleptanalgesia, 101
neuromuscular blocking agent, 26
neuromuscular junction, 18, 123
nightmares, 37
nitric oxide, 22
nitrogen dioxide, 22
nitrous oxide, 21, **22**ff, 38, 61
  effects of, 75, 76
  partial pressure of, 22ff
  sensitivity to, 70
noradrenaline, 25, *see also* Catecholamines
nose, 19
  bleeding, see Epistaxis

occlusion (dental), 131
oedema
  ankle, 5
  general, 9
  laryngeal, 122
oil–gas distribution coefficient, 21
opiates, 11, 90, 103
opium, 79, 103
oral airways, 129
outpatients, 90
overdosage, 33, 140
oxygen
  availability of, 30–1
  concentration, 26
  in an emergency, 58, 130–40
  failure alarm, 64–6
  Hb dissociation curve, 29–31
  maintenance of, 29
  override, 70
  partial pressure of, 29ff
  reserve supply of, 129, 130
  uptake and transport of, 5, 7, **29**ff

packs, 54, 92, 102, 107
pancuronium, 126
papaveretum, 103, 104
paradoxical respiration, 47, 131
partial pressure, 16ff, 21, *see also relevant gases*
pathological problems, **5**ff
patient assessment, 1ff
patient referral, 1

INDEX

pentazocine, 101
pentobarbitone, 98
peripheral vascular resistance, 5, 139
perspiration, 49
pethidine, 98, 103, 104
pH, see Blood
pharynx, 19
phencyclidine, 37
phenothiazine, 96, 104, 105, 128
phenylketonuria, 9
phonation, 131
physical handicap, 10, 11
physiology, problems of, **3ff**
Pierre Robin syndrome, 119
pituitary gland, 9
pneumonitis, 103, 140
porphyria, 88
positions of anaesthesia, see Anaesthesia
potassium, 124
potency, see Anaesthetic
pregnancy, **3**
premedication
  administration, 105
  in children, 106
  narcotic, 89
  with ketamine, 90
pressure
  ambient, 21
  gauge, 23, 63
  partial, see Partial pressure
Priestley, Joseph, 22
procaine, 143
promethazine, 96, 141
propanidid, 36, 89, 99
propranolol, 139
proprioceptors, 49
props, 85, 91
propylene glycol, 36, 102
pseudo-cholinesterase, 124, 142
psychiatric patients, 73
psychological problems, 4
pulse, 129
pyrexia, 7

quantiflex, 70, 71, 75

receptors
  baro, 129
  respiratory, 134
  stretch, 17, 47
recovery, 34, 57

recovery facilities, 58
recumbent position, 41
redistribution, see Drugs
reflexes
  suppression of, 40, 68
  see also Eyelash, laryngeal, vomiting
regurgitation, 4, 41, 139
relative analgesia (RA), **68ff**
  flow rates in, 75
  planes of, 69
  preparation for, **73**
  stage of, 39
relaxation, 20
renal, see Kidney
respiration
  accessory muscles of, 47
  arrest of, 136
  artificial, 51
  collapse of, 81, 140
  depression of, 20, 24, 26, 85
  disorders of, 6, 7, 73
  muscles of, 18, 47
  paradoxical, 47
  physiology of, 19ff
  rate of, 19, 25, 40, 77
  regular, 53
  spontaneous, 40
respiratory acidosis, 137
respiratory centre, 17ff, 25, 47
respiratory tract
  anatomy of, 45
  infection of, 6, 44, 130
resuscitation, 137
resuscitator bag, 129, 134
retrognathia, 130
rheumatoid arthritis, 118
rotameter, 16, 63, 66

salbutamol, 52, 134
second-gas effect, 20
sedation
  in children, 94
  inhalational, **68ff**
  intravenous, **97ff**
  oral, **95ff**
  with local anaesthesia, 2, 13
sedative
  agents, 68, 93
  effect, 68
  oral, 93
see-saw respiration, 47, 131
Sellick's manoeuvre, 41
shivering, 25

INDEX

shock, 33
sickle cell disorders, 7, 8
sniffing-the-morning-air, 117, 118
sodium bicarbonate, 129, 137
spastics, 10, 100
starvation, 13, 14
steroids, 11, 128
stretch receptor, 17, 47
stridor, see Laryngospasm
suction, 92, 112, 113, 129
supersensitivity, 140
supine position, 41, 81, 138
suxamethonium, 123ff
   reactions to, 10, 142
swelling, 12 (see also Oedema)

tachycardia, 9
tactile receptor, 17
temazepam, **95**
temporomandibular joint, 11, 118
   dislocation of, 143
tendon, biceps, 83, 143
tetany, 137
thalassaemia, 8
therapeutic dose (TD), 80
therapeutic index, 80, 88, see also relevant drugs
thiopentone, **34**ff, 87, 115, 140, 142
thoracic cavity, 19
thrombocytopoenia, 8
thrombophlebitis, 36, 99
thrombosis, 79
thymol, 24
thyroid, disorders of, 8, 9
tidal volume, 19, 77
tissuing, 83, 142
tongue, large, see Macroglossia
toxic effects, 9
trachea, 19
tracheostomy, 133
tracheotome, 129
tranquillizers, 103
treatment aids, 2
treatment planning, 12ff, 78
tremor, 36
Trendelenburg position, 74, 81, 138
trichloroethylene, 21, 28
triclofos, 97
tricyclic antidepressants, 11
trigeminal neuralgia, 28

trimeprazine, 96
trismus, 12, 118
tubocurarine, 125

urea, 34
urine, 33, see also Bladder

valve
   air-mixer, 72
   expiratory, 50, 73, 131
   needle, 16, 63, 66
   reducing, 23
   sleeve, 24, 63
vaporization, latent heat of, 23
vaporizer, 16, 20, 24, 63
vapour pressure, 23–9
vascular resistance, 5, 27
vasoconstrictor, 26
vein
   basilic, 82
   cephalic, 82
   in hand, 81
   median, 82
venepuncture, **81**ff, 142
venous return, 4, 41, 82
ventilation, 9, 17, 48
   mechanical, 27, 108
   mechanics of, 19, 47
ventilator, 108
ventricle, 20
ventricular fibrillation, 137
Venturi effect, 67
vocal cords, 6, **115**ff
   granulomas of, 121
vomiting, 10, 14, 28, 68, **139**
   postoperative, 38
Von Willebrand's disease, 12

water, 9
Wells, Horace, 22
wheeze, 49
Wren, Sir Christopher, 79

Yankauer suction end, 134